IIFYM & FLEXIBLE DIETING

Beginners Step-By-Step

"If It Fits Your Macros"

Diet Guide – Quickly &

Easily Lose Weight And

Burn Fat By Counting

Your Macros

By *Jennifer Louissa*

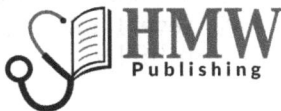

HMW Publishing

For more great books visit:

HMWPublishing.com

Download another book for Free

I want to thank you for purchasing this book and offer you another book (just as long and valuable as this book), "7 Fitness Mistakes You Don't Know You're Making", completely free.

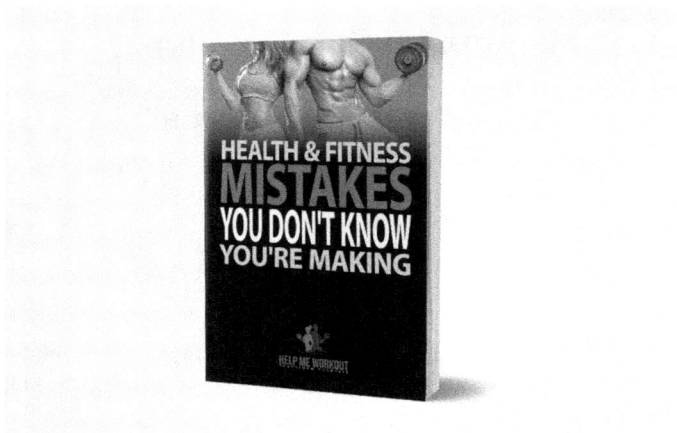

Click the link below to signup and receive it:

www.hmwpublishing.com/gift

In this book, I will break down 7 of the most common fitness mistakes, some of you are probably committing, and I will reveal how you can easily get in the best shape of your life!

In addition to the *7 Fitness Mistakes* book, you will also have an opportunity to get our new books for free, enter giveaways, and receive other valuable emails from me. Again, here is the link to sign up:

www.hmwpublishing.com/gift

TABLE OF CONTENTS

Introduction

I want to thank you and congratulate you for purchasing the "IFYM Flexible Dieting & Counting Macros" book. The best fat loss *strategy*, in my experience, has been IIFYM (If It Fits Your Macros). Another name for this revolutionary way of eating is *Flexible Dieting* or simply *Counting Your Macros*. IIFYM has been used for years now. Both people who aim to lose fat or build muscle use it.

IIFYM & Flexible Dieting offers anyone the opportunity to tailor their diets to their favourite nutritious foods, mixing their favourite treats every day, and still make progress towards their fitness goals.

Is it realistic to say that you're never going to eat ice cream, burgers or pizza again? Are your only carbs going to come from veggies (I can't even stand the thought)? Are you going to trade all these so-called "dirty foods" out for meals consisting of chicken, brown rice, broccoli and maybe some sweet potatoes if you're lucky? My guess is probably not. That approach to weight loss can cause you to have a total binge day in the future. Not only would your diet be strict and boring, but you'll most likely gain back all the "strict diet" weight you lost in the first place.

IIFYM is also a method of dieting used to improve body composition by tracking macronutrients (macros). Three main macros are traditionally accounted for: protein, carbs, and fats. By monitoring macros, you naturally track your calories as well.

This way of dieting has been gaining vast popularity and chances are you've heard of it. If you've done any research on IIFYM & Flexible Dieting in the past you've, perhaps, realized that no foods are off limits. No food groups are labeled good or bad for you. What matters, in this style of dieting, is if your macro budget has room for the foods you want to eat. If so then you're in the clear, but more on that soon.

So how did this type of dieting come about? Well, bodybuilder's in the old days simply got tired of eating the same bland foods when preparing for a competition. They ate the kind of food that scares people away from attempting to lose weight in the first place! These boring, clean meals, included chicken, broccoli, rice, veggies, eggs, and well—you get the picture. There's no denying that this *"bro science"* approach to dieting works, but the real question is: is it worth it? After years of making bodybuilders miserable If It Fits Your Macros was born. IIFYM is thus a way to improve one's body composition by not solely relying on clean foods. Thanks again for purchasing this book, I hope you enjoy it and please don't forget to leave us an honest review!

Also, before you get started, I recommend you joining our email newsletter to receive updates on any upcoming new book releases or promotions. You can sign-up for free, and as a bonus, you will receive a free gift. Our *"Health & Fitness Mistakes*

You Don't Know You're Making" book! This book has been written to demystify, expose the top do's and don'ts and to finally equip you with the information you need to get in the best shape of your life. Due to the overwhelming amount of mis-information and lies told by magazines and self-proclaimed "gurus", it's becoming harder and harder to get reliable information to get in shape. As opposed to having to go through dozens of biased, unreliable and un-trustworthy sources to get your health & fitness information. Everything you need to help you has been broken down in this book for you to easily follow and to immediately get results to achieve your desired fitness goals in the shortest amount of time.

Once again, to join our free email newsletter and to receive a free copy of this valuable book, please visit the link and signup now: www.hmwpublishing.com/gift

CHAPTER 1: WHAT IS "IIFYM"?

A common misconception of IIFYM (If It Fits Your Macros) is that it's just an excuse to eat junk food every day. This is not the case. Contrary to popular belief, IIFYM is not about eating pop tarts for breakfast every day. Unlike traditional diets, you have the *option* to eat what you want, when you want, if you make it fit into your eating plans.

Although the option to eat so-called greasy foods (pizza, burgers, ice cream, cookies, etc.) exists, you certainly don't have to part take in it. The edge that IIFYM dieting has over traditional dieting is its flexibility. This flexibility offers you the ability to improve your body composition without having to be perfect or strict with your diet behaviour.

There's no reason to be super strict or go on a fad diet. The fad diet approach never last and there seems to be one coming out every other month! Specifically, there's no need for dramatic, and unhealthy, calorie restrictions or any elimination of any particular macronutrient (this includes low-carb approaches). Once you understand the fundamentals of calories and macros, you'll have a better understanding of why hardcore and fad diets fall short.

Although IIFYM can be used for gaining lean muscle mass, *IIFYM: The Ultimate Beginner's Guide* is tailored towards implementing IIFYM for fat loss. This style of eating is more realistic for people who want to lose fat and enjoy the process.

The benefits of IIFYM:

- Realistic & psychologically beneficial;
- A long-term approach a healthy lifestyle:
- Compatible with the energy balance law (more on this in Chapter 2).
- Flexible food choices;
- It works perfectly with My Fitness Pal (IIFYM-friendly smartphone app).

This approach to fat loss is centered around knowing your macros and hitting your daily macro goals.

My Fitness Pal is the number one tool that makes IIFYM easy to implement.

The following chapters are the fundamentals that you'll need to know to integrate IIFYM into your daily routine.

CHAPTER 2: DEBUNKING THE MYTHS

As with anything new and different, there are going to be pros and cons as well as many misconceptions – and a few distorted myths. In this chapter, we're going to sort those out so the truth will shine through.

Debunking Myth #1: You can gorge on junk food and lose weight.

The flexible dieting plan is an inclusive plan. You will not be told to abstain from any specific food groups. Because of this surprising (and different) concept, the myth is that a person can eat all the junk food they want, which of course is entirely erroneous.

Let's go back and refer to your personal goals. Do you want to achieve:

- Weight loss?

- Weight maintenance?

- Muscle toning?

- Muscle building?

Common sense says if you want to build muscles, it's not going to happen on a steady diet of ice cream and chocolate chip cookies. Plus the fact that fiber is missing.

This myth may have emerged due to online blogs, articles, and ads that have to do with flexible dieting. What's the most common graphics featured on those sites? Donuts, candy, pizza, and maybe a Big Mac.

The reason for this is because it indeed is good news that a diet no longer has to be torture and agony. After all, if you can improve your body composition while still enjoying some junk food, let's tell the world – even if it has to involve lots of junk food pictures.

But let's return to reality. Flexible dieters eat a diet composed of whole food sources with a dash of fun indulgences on the side. The wise, flexible dieter still makes it a goal to hit their daily macronutrient intakes because health is always important.

Debunking Myth #2:

Clean foods are the only healthy foods so flexible dieting cannot be healthy.

Granted a great deal of the American diet is made up of processed foods, some of which are not indeed food at all but simply manufactured products that have little nutritional value. However, to get caught up in the fallacy that *clean foods* are the only *healthy foods* merely is another trap.

To follow that line of thinking we have to return to the excellent food vs. bad food mentality. What good can ever come out of making certain foods *off-limits?* Because the moment you give in to temptation and eat foods that are on the no-no list, the guilt issues resurface. And who needs those?

Various studies have shown that just as soon as a particular food is restricted, the desire for it grows. Even if that person never really had a craving for that food before the restriction. Difficult to explain, but it's true. We are psychological beings, and this is how the human mind (and emotions) operates.

Debunking Myth #3:

Flexible diets lack structure

(they're all over the place).

This myth is quite easily explained. It merely arises because habitual dieters are so accustomed to the shackles of a restricted diet. They have confused limitations with structure. They're not the same.

Indeed, flexible dieting is a structured method, but without the restraints and restrictions. The successful flexible dieter will take the time to consider what food source – and in what amount –

is the best for the activities of this day. Tomorrow may be different.

Debunking Myth #4:

Flexible dieters are looking for an easy way out – they're lazy.

This fourth and final myth, to me, is the most humorous. To follow the logic of this thinking, one has to assume that jumping from one restrictive fad diet to another while trying to remember which foods are restricted on which diet, while excitedly awaiting the Saturday night cheat meal, is considered a productive way to spend your time. I don't think so.

It does require a good deal of planning for the flexible dieter to find the foods that fit with their daily macronutrients. The difference here is that you are thinking for yourself, rather than having some diet guru tell you how to make it work for you. You may want to learn more about nutrition, food, and macronutrients. Your incentive will be stronger, simply because you're not entering the dieter's torture chamber. You're discovering what's best for you and your goals.

In the next chapter we're going to do just that – take a closer look at macronutrients.

CHAPTER 3: FLEXIBLE DIETING VS. STRICT DIETING

In this chapter, we want to take a close look at how the typical strict diets/fad diets compare to the flexible dieting method. We want to look at three separate areas:

- 1) Body.

- 2) Mind (emotions).

- 3) Lifestyle.

1) Comparison of Your Body:

Strict / Fad Diets

Dieters who have spent years on the fad-dieting roller coaster often cease to appreciate the complexity of their body and how it functions. Misplaced priorities put many aspects of health and wellness on the back burner. This means that the body can be abused and health can be compromised in the quest for that *perfect* body weight. (As mentioned earlier, *perfection* is impossible to attain.)

The stopping and starting of various types of diets put stress on the digestive system, as well as vital organs such as the heart and liver.

Likewise, switching restrictive diets can also be harmful. This happens when a discouraged dieter moves from one diet to another in search of the secret to weight loss. Diets that forbid one or more food groups can cause nutritional deficiencies and throw the body entirely out of whack.

Another dangerous effect on chronic dieters is the increased inability to recognize the body's signals of hunger and fullness. Those who suffer from this *dieting side effect* report that they can go for long periods of time without any sense of being hungry. But then, once they start eating again, their appetite goes entirely out of control.

By its very essence, the fad diet is an on-again, off-again pattern, which as mentioned, creates some hardships on overall health.

Flexible Diet

The flexible diet can hardly even be called a diet. In direct contrast to fad diets, this points to a *lifestyle* rather than a quick fix. This means less stress on the body and the body's systems.

Remember we stressed that the flexible diet starts with *your* goals and purposes, not just some one-size-fits-all type of diet.

So what is your goals? Is it:

. Weight loss?

. Weight maintenance?

. Muscle toning?

. Muscle building?

Whichever it is, this is where you begin. From there you move into which foods best work to achieve these goals. If you get most of your daily calories (let's say 80%) from mostly unprocessed, nutrient-dense foods, then with the flexible diet you can feel free to fill the remaining 20% with the indulgences that you love. (Ice cream? Pizza? Chocolate chip cookies?) The key is to know how many calories you can *afford* for that day and stay within that range.

Now you can be as lean and healthy as you want just by using the flexible diet method. No more guilt, no more stress, no more dieting failures. Your body can rest from the yo-yo, back-and-forth torture of strict dieting.

Your mind can rest as well. And that brings us to our next point.

2) Comparison of Your Mind:

Strict / Fad Diets

People who are involved in the sales industry have a saying:

"The confused mind always says no."

To a salesperson, that means you must stay focused and keeps things simple. Compare this to the world of strict dieting. Did you ever enter a world that was so filled with vague terms, conflicting suppositions, and confusing information? The world of dieting and weight loss is rife with all of the above. You talk to one person who is on a specific diet, and they firmly believe that everything they are doing (down to the last stalk of celery) is the right way to go about things.

Talk to another person who is on yet another type of diet, and they are just as convinced and religious about their approach.

That is until they are either 1) miserable and bored with the whole mess, or 2) they hear about yet another diet that seems much better and more efficient than the one they're on at the moment.

Confusion reigns! And the confused mind always says no.

Confusion equates to a lack of confidence, and a lack of confidence relates to a lack of commitment. And since both of these individuals are miserable anyway, quitting becomes all that much more comfortable.

The mind and the emotions have a great deal to do with the process of weight loss. The most significant culprit in this area is guilt. Because most diets are a setup for failure, the chronic dieter is all too familiar with the agony of failing – time after time. If any success is involved – and it sometimes is – it's short-lived.

Instead of food simply being *food*, it has been transformed into an *enemy* that must be conquered. Dieters become exhausted just thinking about diet and weight loss and all the anxiety that is involved. Many times this can lead to the person seeing themselves as a loser and a failure. One who is "less than." Many begin to give up – not just on a diet but *self* as well. Depression is often the result.

Are these types of consequences worth it?

Have you ever heard of stair-step dieting? Perhaps you've experienced it, but had no name for it. What happens is this:

The dieter goes on a diet and successfully loses weight. Later that weight is gained back and *then some*. If this happens repeatedly, the accumulated effect is continued weight gain. With it comes the shame and a state of emotional turmoil which can end up in bingeing cycles. The feeling is that they failed simply because they didn't try hard enough, or didn't have enough willpower, or didn't have what it takes to stick with it.

Again, it's a setup for failure.

Flexible Dieting

None of the above is applicable when it comes to *flexible dieting*. The roller coaster cycle of moving from diet to diet is broken once and for all. Because you're eating what's right for you, eating your food preferences, eating foods you enjoy, the dieting-misery is out of the picture altogether. Guilt and shame are also removed.

Food becomes food again – that's as it's supposed to be in life. No longer are you in a battle with the very substance that's needed to sustain you and your health. This brings a fantastic amount of rest, peace, and freedom.

Eating the foods that are right for you and your goals and purposes, and moving away from the stress, guilt, and shame can add years to your life. As we are all aware, stress can be a silent killer, so why give it an extra place in your life over dieting?

Here's the uptake. Eat foods you like and enjoy. Balance your macronutrient intake. Restrict calories – but only moderately. Like magic, the psychological burden of trying to lose weight is gone. In fact, losing weight becomes comfortable and enjoyable. Sounds like something a person could live with for a sustained length of time, right?

Does that mean you'll never slip up? Well, you're human, aren't you? You go out to eat with friends, and you eat more than usual. Just go with the flow. No need to suffer through guilt and shame. Just work it (the possibility of occasional slip-ups) into your plan and don't fear it. (No more beating yourself up!)

Your calorie deficiency may have moved over into a calorie surplus. A modest binge is not the end of the world. Just get back on track and carry on.

If you're one who's been chained to the dieting cycle, does this sound like a different way of life?

You're right. So next, let's look at *lifestyle.*

3) Comparison of Your Lifestyle:

Strict / Fad Diets

The lifestyle of the habitual dieter who uses the strict dieting plans is neither pleasant nor appealing. It's a life filled with fretting and worrying, mixed in with bouts of failure, hopelessness, and discouragement.

The person caught in this trap is just that – trapped; hence, the cycles have continued for so long, and it's difficult to envision getting free of them.

The unsuccessful dieter is usually not a very happy person. In fact, many are just plain old miserable. What kind of life is that? It's not good for the one who's trying to lose weight, and it's probably not a whole lot of fun for those who are in proximity. (That would be friends, family, acquaintances, and co-workers.) What's more boring than to hear the weeping and moaning over the latest diet failure?

Flexible Dieting

Compare this with the lifestyle of the one who has discovered the flexible dieting method. This person is allowed to go to a company dinner and not sit there and fret that their current diet does not approve everything on the *menu*. Not at all. This person can relax because she knows her macronutrient intake for the day and knows exactly what she can eat, or not eat and still be on track for meeting her goals.

This person is stress-free (no whining or complaining) and is quite enjoyable to be around.

The flexible dieting method *becomes a lifestyle*. It's a plan that can be maintained for months – and then for years. No set up for failure here. No falling off the wagon.

As you can see from what has been covered in this chapter, the differences between the strict (fad) diet and the flexible diet are many. In the next section, we want to filter out some of the myths about flexible dieting. Having the full, clear picture is essential.

CHAPTER 4: THE FUNDAMENTALS OF CALORIES

"Everything is energy, and that's all there is to it. Match the frequency of the reality you want, and you cannot help but get that reality. It can be no other way. This is not philosophy. This is physics."
– *Albert Einstein*

Weight loss is derived from universal laws at its core. There's one law in particular that explains how we lose weight. The body obeys the first law of thermodynamics. The first rule simply states that energy can neither be created nor destroyed and is often referred to as the energy balance equation (or energy balance law).

$$\Delta U = Q - W$$

(Change in Internal Energy) =

(Heat) - (Work)

This law gets the credit for how much weight we lose or gain.

A calorie, by definition, is a unit of heat energy.

If you eat more than your body requires every day, you're bound to gain weight. Gaining weight typically means the body is a **caloric surplus**. Unwanted fat stores are attributed to the excess intake of these, hopefully, delicious units of energy.

If you eat less than your body needs every day, you're going to lose weight. Losing weight is attributed to being in a **caloric deficit**.

Our bodies can also be at equilibrium, meaning our weight remains the same. In this case, the body is at a **caloric maintenance** level.

Does this mean that you can eat whatever you want while in a caloric deficit and still lose weight? Yes, it's possible but ill-advised. People who try this usually neglect specific macronutrient nourishment, which we'll discuss in more detail later on in this book.

The focus of this book is on losing weight, specifically from fat, while being in a caloric deficit and not in misery at the same time!

When the energy balance equation is applied to fitness, it simply translates to energy (foods) that enters the body and strength that leaves the body as either work (exercise) or heat.

$$\Delta E = E_{in} - E_{out}$$

(Change in Body Weight) = (Energy Consumed) - (Energy Expended)

I'm of the opinion that weight should come off as fast as possible! I don't want to be guessing (eyeballing portions) and hoping I'm in a caloric deficit. I've tried that approach (the eating clean foods approach) to weight loss, and I can confirm it's a drag. There's no need to drag out the weight loss process. That approach to weight loss usually leads to people quitting because of a mix of frustration and disappointing progress.

I know one thing for certain: numbers don't lie.

A usual concern for people starting IIFYM is thinking about numbers or math. IIFYM only requires algebra gymnastics if you don't take advantage of IIFYM-friendly apps. Food tracking apps like "MyFitnessPal" (MFP) have been created to make tracking food consumption a breeze. MFP does all the heavy lifting (the math) for you! Here's an example:

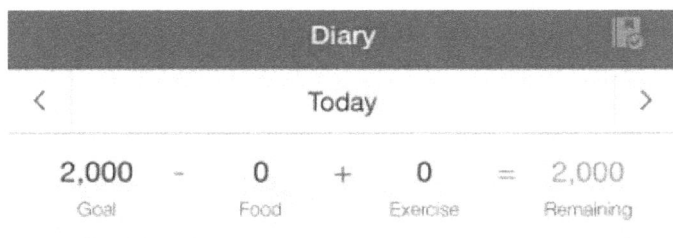

		Diary				
<			Today			>
2,000	-	0	+	0	=	2,000
Goal		Food		Exercise		Remaining

Look familiar? It's the energy balance equation in action slightly rearranged.

The easiest way to start IIFYM is by logging in what you eat with MFP. If you choose to you can track your exercise as well!

We'll be using MFP as our food tracker because it's the most highly rated and popular food tracking app available. Think of this app as the fuel gauge in your car. You wouldn't want to go on a road trip from California to Washington with your fuel gauge broken. You might make it to your destination, but you will encounter a variety of unnecessary obstacles along the way.

Knowing how much fuel is in the "tank" is imperative to losing weight promptly. MFP will be your energy fuel gauge. This handy app will give you an insight into why you're getting closer or further to your goal. Knowing your total calorie consumption carries the potential to save you time on your journey. In other words, it eliminates guessing and if you value time as I do then guessing is something you do not want to be associated with.

MFP can be used on any smart device (iPhone, Android, iPad/tablet, or on a regular computer). Most people use their smartphones to track their food intake because it's the most convenient option, namely because your phone's camera can be a barcode scanner.

I'll be showing you step-by-step examples of how to track your food, and thus your macros, on an iPhone (MFP's user interface is similar and consistent across all smart devices). Before we get started, it's time for you to take your first action step!

Out Your Body's Daily Calorie Requirement

In addition to knowing about calories, the flexible dieter will know their macronutrient requirement in relation to their height, weight, and activity level.

Once you know your body's daily calorie requirements, the next step is relatively clear-cut:

. Eat more calories = weight gain.

- Eat fewer calories = weight loss.

- Eat this amount of calories = weight maintenance.

Why Each Main Macronutrient Matters

Before we leave this tutorial on how to calculate your macros, let's take a closer look at each of the three macronutrients and why they are essential:

Carbohydrates

We need carbohydrates because:

- They are the body's primary source of fuel.

- Can be easily used by the body for energy.

- Provide glucose which is used by tissues and cells in the body for energy.

- The central nervous system, kidneys, brain and muscles (including the heart) must have carbohydrates to function properly.

. Carbs are essential for intestinal health and waste elimination.

Protein:

We need protein for:

. Growth (especially significant for children, teens, and pregnant women).

. Tissue repair.

. Proper functioning of the immune system.

. Producing essential hormones and enzymes inside the body.

. Energy when carbohydrates are not available.

. Preserving lean muscle mass.

Fats:

Fats are not the culprits most diet gurus make them out to be. In fact, good fats are needed for survival, and at least 20-35% of calories should come from good fat sources. Fats are necessary for:

. Allowing healthy growth and development.

. Providing the most concentrated source of energy to the body.

. Helping the body absorb essential vitamins such as A, D, E, K and carotenoids.

. Providing cushioning for internal organs.

. Maintaining cell membranes.

. Providing taste, consistency, and stability of foods.

A quick glance at these lists gives substance to the fact that we all need a wide variety of foods to maintain good health. By their very nature, restrictive diets will eliminate one or more of these health benefits.

In addition to the macronutrients, remember the body also needs a healthy amount of water each day and added micronutrients. Micronutrients are the trace vitamins and minerals that round out a healthy diet.

Cardio:

So, to get the body of your dreams, do you need to partake in hours of mind-numbing cardio such as walking on the treadmill or stair climbing?

The answer to the above question is: probably not.

The primary purpose of the aerobic exercise is to increase the heart rate to burn more calories. If excess calories are not consumed, then cardio is not required, it is that simple – many professional bodybuilders are so precise with their caloric intake that they can obtain a competition level physique (3-4% body fat with masses of lean muscle) just through diet manipulation alone!

If you do, however, surpass your caloric target for the day, then cardio can be a convenient tool to offset these excess calories. But don't forget "you can't out train a bad diet." If you calculate your calories using this method, I will present to you further in this book that you will not be required to do any cardio.

I personally incorporate small amounts of cardio (in the form of high intensity intervals) into my routine to lose the last few pounds of fat instead of dropping my calories lower once I have recalculated my TDEE. TDEE and calculations will be discussed a bit later on in this book.

Note: aerobic activities are fantastic for cardiovascular health, increasing performance in sports, speed, and agility, etc. However, that is outside the scope of this book.

Calories:

So what is a calorie?

A calorie is an energy source. Humans require calories to maintain life. We are continually trying to increase and decrease our caloric intake based on our goals, such as: whether we want to slim down, gain lean muscle mass or perform a particular way of sports. If a calorie that is consumed is not utilized, it will be converted by the body and stored as fat.

Calories can come from several different macronutrient sources. These include:

- **Protein** – 4 calories per gram– protein serves as building blocks for lean muscle mass.

- **Carbohydrates** – 4 calories per gram – our bodies use carbohydrates as the primary energy source. Carbohydrates are broken down into 2 subcategories (both contain 4 cals/gram).

- **Simple carbohydrates** – these are the sugary processed carbohydrates that are found in foods such as lollies, chocolate, and fruit. Simple carbohydrates are absorbed quickly and cause a large insulin spike.

- **Complex carbohydrates** – These carbohydrates are the 'clean' slow digesting carbohydrates that are known for sustained energy. Complex carbs are found in brown rice, sweet potato, and oats.

- **Fat** – 9 calories per gram – Healthy fats are vital for bodily functions such as hormone levels. Fats are also broken down into several categories:

- **Saturated fat** – found in dairy and meat, can raise cholesterol.

- **Unsaturated fat** – found in vegetable oils, used to lower cholesterol.

- **Alcohol** – 7 calories per gram – empty calories (alcohol does not contain any macronutrients).

Calculating Your Macronutrients

To begin your flexible diet, you need to know your daily caloric goal! Be sure to have a calculator or degree in mathematics on hand. To calculate this goal, the following formula is used (please note the slight variation in the formula for men and women):

Based on the extremely accurate Mifflin - St Jeor equation

- MEN: BMR = [9.99 x weight (kg)] + [6.25 x height (cm)] - [4.92 x age (years)] + 5

  WOMEN: BMR = [9.99 x weight (kg)] + [6.25 x height (cm)] - [4.92 x age (years)] -161

The above equation will give you your BMR – this is your Basal Metabolic Rate. In other words, the number of calories your body needs to function while at rest.

You then multiply the BMR by an 'activity variable' to obtain your TDEE (total daily energy expenditure). This Activity Factor is the cost of living, and it is based on more than just your workouts. It also includes work/lifestyle, sports and the thermogenic effect of food (necessarily the amount of energy burned in the process of digesting food).

Average activity variables are as follows:

- 1.2 = Sedentary - Little or no exercise + desk job

- 1.3-1.4 = Lightly Active - Little daily activity and light exercise 1-3 days a week

- 1.5-1.6 = Moderately Active - Moderately active daily life and moderate exercise 3-5 days a week

- 1.7-1.8 = Very Active - Physically demanding lifestyle and hard training or sports 6-7 days a week

- 1.9-2.0 = Extremely Active - Hard daily exercise or sports and physical job

Below are some examples of this calculation performed correctly:

Male

- 90kg male – 21 years old - 187cm tall – desk job, minimal exercise

- $[9.99 \times 90] + [6.25 \times 187] - [4.92 \times 21] - 5$ Activity Level 1.2 = 2350 calories

- 70kg male – 18 years old - 170cm tall – physical job, lots of exercise

- $[9.99 \times 70] + [6.25 \times 170] - [4.92 \times 18] - 5$ Activity level 1.7 = 2852 calories

Female

- 65kg female – 28 years old – 140cm – desk
  job, minimal exercise

  [9.99 65] + [6.25 140] – [4.92 28] – 161

  Activity level 1.2 = 1500 calories

- 55kg female – 18 years old – 150cm –
  moderately active

  [9.99 55] + [6.25 150] – [4.92 18] – 161

  Activity level 1.5 = 1414 calories

Alternatively, you can use an online calculator
based on the Mifflin – St Jeor equation, merely
googling *"Mifflin st jeor equation calculator"* will
result in several online calculators.

CHAPTER 5: GOAL-BASED CALORIE CONSUMPTION

Now that you have calculated your TDEE (Total Daily Energy Expenditure), you need to determine what your goal is. Do you want to maintain your current state? Do you want to strip fat? Do you want to pack on lean muscle?

The most significant mistake being made when deciding to lose weight is to go into starvation or 'crash' diet. Dropping to 1000~ calories per day will initially give you a period of weight loss at an impressive rate, however. This WILL cause metabolic damage (the process of your body rapidly decreasing its metabolism and the rate at which calories are burned due to the minimal amount of food it is receiving, mostly going into survival mode). Also, you guessed it: the only way to repair a damaged metabolism is to start to eat more slowly. Crash dieting is not sustainable - do not do it.

- For weight loss – consume 500 calories below your TDEE per day.

- For lean muscle gain – consume 500 calories above your TDEE per day.

- To maintain – consume the exact number of calories as your TDEE each day.

As your progress begins to slow down, it is time to re-calculate your TDEE via the same formula you used previously (listed above) as you will now find that your TDEE has changed! As you add lean mass, your TDEE will considerably increase. As you begin to lose weight, you will notice your TDEE has decreased (and, therefore, after a month you only be eating 200 calories under your TDEE instead of the 500 calories that you were initially consuming under).

Note: I personally recalculate TDEE on a monthly basis; I recommend you do the same.

Calorie Macronutrient Breakdown:

Now that we have determined your calorie goal, and established that you could eat whichever foods you choose to reach this magical caloric value, it is essential to develop an accurate ratio of protein, carbohydrates, and fats to consume.

For optimal performance in sports and resistance training (as well as to keep your appetite in check), I recommend consuming at least 30% of your daily calories from protein, with the remaining 70% coming from a breakdown of calories and fats.

You'll notice in the standard macronutrient splits listed below, the percentage of calories derived from fat does not drop below 20%. This is because hormones are constructed from cholesterol along with other fat molecules; decreasing the rate of fat consumed any lower can suppress your healthy hormone levels. Why is this an issue, you ask? Because these hormones drive the growth and development of your body, your metabolism, reproduction system, and mood. Low fat intake causes a deficiency in essential fatty acids and also highly increases your risk of cancer.

Although, as stated, you will lose fat by merely consuming under your TDEE calories and gain weight by eating above your TDEE, I would highly recommend following a high protein approach. If you neglect your protein intake, you will not build and retain lean muscle. Meals high in protein will also keep you feeling fuller for longer, unlike those rich in carbohydrates and fats.

Note: When referring to a macronutrient breakdown, the order listed is Protein: Carbohydrates: Fat

Common macronutrient splits include:

30P:50C:20F

moderately high protein, high carbohydrate, low fat.

Often used when going through a mass building or 'bulking' phase.

35P:40C:30F

Moderately high protein, moderately high carbohydrates, higher fats than usual. This is a reasonably even split of macronutrients, and I would recommend this style of macronutrient split when maintaining your current body composition.

40P:40C:20F

High protein, high carbohydrates, and low fat.The most commonly used macronutrient split used by bodybuilders and fitness enthusiasts today, used for both fat loss and addition of lean muscle mass by merely adjusting the number of calories consumed.

50P:30C:20F

High protein, low carbohydrate, low fat.

This macronutrient split is often used for ongoing fat loss diets, as the high protein content keeps the individual feeling quite full and content between their meals. With this low level of carbohydrates, refeeds are necessary (this will be discussed further in the book).

35P:60C:5F

Moderate protein, high fat, minimal carbohydrates.

A diet comprised of these macronutrients is known as a 'ketogenic diet.' The primary purpose of this diet is to adjust the body to use fat as the primary stored energy source as opposed to carbohydrates – when the body enters this state (which takes several days), it is in a state of ketosis. I would not recommend following this style of macronutrient breakdown due to the previously mentioned hormone suppression that occurs with low-fat diets. Food choice is also insufficient to essentially meats, nuts and a small portion of vegetables, which defeats the purpose of flexible dieting.

Personal Note:

I follow a 40:35:25 macronutrient breakdown.

For example – I am currently consuming 2800 calories to trim the last bit of body fat; my daily macronutrient breakdown is 280 grams of protein per day, 245 grams of carbohydrates per day and 78 grams of fats per day.

Required Macronutrients:

Fiber

Fiber is an essential macronutrient that our body needs for aiding digestion. A 'clean eating' diet comprises lots of foods that contain high fiber content – however, while flexible dieting, it is equally essential that we meet our fiber needs.

Women need to aim for 22 – 28 grams of dietary fiber per day.

Men need to aim for 28 – 34 grams of dietary fiber per day.

There is a range of fiber supplements available on the market. However, these are (as the name suggests) only a supplement to your regular fiber intake. Foods high in fiber include whole grains, fruits, and vegetables (note: these are all forms of carbohydrates).

Refeeds

What is a Refeed?

If you are embarking on a fat loss journey through the use of flexible dieting (or any style of dieting!), it is paramount to incorporate structured refeeds. Please note that this section is irrelevant if you intend to follow a calorie surplus to gain lean mass. A structured refeed is a 24-hour period in which you drastically alter your macronutrient breakdown after being in a calorie deficit (consuming fewer calories than your TDEE).

Why is a Refeed Essential?

A refeed will boost your metabolism and assist in restoring your Leptin hormone levels - Leptin is the king of all fat burning hormones. When in a calorie deficit, your metabolism will drop (meaning fewer calories are being burnt), plus your leptin hormone levels will drop in the attempt by the body to spare body fat. This is a safety mechanism put in place for the body.

We need to understand that our body is resistant to change, no matter what our current body composition is - our body does not want to change. The human body does not want to lose fat; it simply wants to survive. Consuming below your TDEE (Total Daily Energy Expenditure) will force your body to slow down your metabolism, resulting in a lower caloric intake to continually burn body fat.

As the metabolism begins to slow and Leptin levels drop, it becomes a lot harder to burn excess body fat. Therefore, including a refeed day into your diet will encourage your body to burn fat at a consistent rate.

The leaner you are, the more often you will need to refeed; lower body fat = lower leptin levels. This is based on body fat percentage; you will learn how to calculate this in the section below.

Body fat Percentage	Frequency of Refeed
Over 20%	Monthly
15 – 20%	Fortnightly
10 – 15%	Weekly
Under 10%	Twice Weekly

Refeed Frequency

Please refer to the following table for refeed timing:

Carbohydrate Intake During a Refeed

On your structured refeed day, I recommend you leave your protein and fat intakes the same as any other day. However, double your carbohydrate intake for this 24 hour period. This will put you slightly over your maintenance calories for the day, but it will have long-term benefits (as discussed above).

Here is an example of my regular caloric intake:

- 2800 calories (500 below my TDEE)

- 280 grams of protein

- 245 grams of carbohydrates

- 78 grams of fats

Here is my typical caloric intake on a structured refeed day:

- 3780 calories (580 calories above my TDEE)

- 280 grams of protein

- 490 grams of carbohydrates

- 78 grams of fats

As we have previously addressed, a carbohydrate is a carbohydrate – you can derive these extra carbohydrates from whichever source you choose, it does not matter whether they are simple or complex. On a refeed day, I typically indulge in oats, ice cream, pancakes, bananas and pasta as these are all very rich in carbohydrates.

CHAPTER 6: MEAL TIMING

I'm sure you've heard this before: to achieve your fitness goals, you need to eat a more significant number of smaller meals (for example 5 – 6 meals a day). This, along with clean eating, is preached heavily by nutritionists and personal trainers.

What if I told you meal frequency and nutrient timing doesn't matter at all? Or that eating 6 times a day will not affect your metabolism or metabolic rate? That you can eat carbs right before bed and you won't gain fat?

Upon first thinking about this, it may sound like I'm making this all up. Surely consuming food before sleeping will be stored as fat as you are not actively exercising to utilize these calories. However, our body does not operate like this – it is continually looking at the bigger picture, the calories/macronutrients we consume over a 24 or 48-hour period. Your body is frequently breaking down and repairing itself, storing and oxidizing nutrients.

It's hard to instantly change your beliefs on an aspect of fitness that is preached continuously, but a paradigm shift is required – individuals spend far too much time stressing over the timing of their meals and how many they consume a day rather than focusing on the most important aspect of dieting.

<u>Eat what you want, when you want - as long as you hit your caloric goal.</u>

A study on the "Effect of the Pattern of Food Intake on Human Energy Metabolism" states:

Lose Fat, Not Weight

Before we delve deeper into the following sections, it is imperative we clarify weight loss and fat loss.

Weight loss is one of the most lucrative topics in existence. The majority of people claim that they want to lose weight or fat, interchangeably switching between both of these hot keywords –

little do they know there is a big difference between the two.

Weight Loss refers to your total body weight; this is the sum of your bones, muscles, organs, water, and fat.

Fat Loss refers to the amount of fat you are carrying on your body, measured as a percentage of your total body weight.

When weight loss is discussed, I'm sure you can now see that this is indeed a reference for people wanting to lose fat. In the 'tracking progress' section below, I will show you how to accurately assess your fat loss progress if this is indeed your goal.

The primary issue when discussing 'weight loss' is how unreliable it is. Your total weight fluctuates daily based upon stomach, bowel and bladder content, water loss and retention; with a large carbohydrate intake, water is bound (this is why a low/no carb diet will initially give you an impressive decrease in weight, as you no longer retain anywhere near as much water). Muscle loss and gain, as well as fat loss and gain, also play a major role. Researchers refer to those who lose weight easily but find it harder to gain weight to be 'spendthrift' with those that can gain weight easily but have more of an issue losing weight to be 'thrifty' – this ties in with the body types.

Sustainability of Flexible Dieting

How sustainable is flexible dieting? Can you continuously eat delicious foods of your choice and consistently make progress?

Of course! Flexible dieting/IIFYM will continue to work as long as you are reaching your calorie/ macronutrient goal and recalculating your TDEE on a regular basis. However, if you intend to follow a flexible dieting approach for an extended period, there are a few points that must be addressed

- Continually deriving your carbohydrates from simple sugars can lead to adverse health conditions, such as increased blood sugar levels (which can lead to diabetes), high blood pressure and more. I regularly have check-ups with my local general practitioner to ensure all my levels are within a healthy, normal range.

- If you do not include a variety of vegetables within your diet, I continue to stress the importance of getting your daily vitamins and minerals via the supplementation of a multivitamin.

- Ensure you are reaching your fiber intake for the day before you consume all of your carbohydrates.

- You should time your meals based on your workout schedule. You should consume a pre-workout meal 60 – 90 minutes before training, comprised of protein and complex carbohydrates for energy. Immediately after your workout is the ideal time to consume simple carbohydrates (chocolate, lollies, etc.) to refuel your glycogen stores (which are now depleted from stressful exercise). You will not make any additional weight loss/gains by doing this. However, for overall energy and recovery pre-and post-workout nutrition are vital.

- The primary purpose of IIFYM is to achieve your desired body composition. It does not emphasize overall heart or organ health, unlike clean eating.

Therefore, from a health perspective, it is worth adapting the theory and principles behind IIFYM into your diet, as opposed to eating sugar ridden lollies as your primary source of carbohydrates.

CHAPTER 7: MFP FEATURES FOR IIFYM SUCCESS

"You'll never change your life until you change something you do daily. The secret of your success is found in your daily routine." – John C. Maxwell

At the end of the day, it's the people who regulate their food intake who have the most significant successes in their fat loss journeys. I don't even consider logging in food a hassle anymore. Once you start seeing progress with IIFYM, the once upon a time "hassle," gets transmuted into a habit.

The price of doing what everyone else does is simple: little to no weight loss progress and return to old habits. Of course, it's easier just to grab some healthy food and cook it, or in some cases, heating up leftovers. This is the approach most people take.

I want you to have long-term success, and to do that, in fitness or any other area of life, it requires obtaining new habits. While reading this chapter, remember that you're learning a process that'll take you to your end goal if you commit.

Saving Time with Meal Entries

When I first started tracking my food I didn't want to think about numbers every time I was going to eat. What I realized was that measuring foods (in ounces, grams, cups, tablespoons etc.) wasn't as bad when you created a meal plan which was tailored just for you, a topic that's coming up soon. Combine a meal plan, with MFP's logging features, and tracking becomes extremely easy.

MFP makes tracking what you eat easily because it upkeeps a history database, similar to an internet browsing history, of the foods you've eaten in the past. Having a database, built into MFP, is great because it quickly retrieves past food entries and allows it to be easily added to any meal you choose.

A great shortcut on MFP is the *Smart Copy* feature which has the potential to remove any hassle from food tracking. The *Smart Copy* feature will save you the most time if you have a meal plan, or consistently eat the same meals every day. It quickly lets you add what you ate yesterday (or X amount of days before) to the present day's corresponding meal. You do this with one quick swipe of a finger.

Take the following steps to enable the *Smart Copy* feature. The steps should also be a great example of how this process looks like.

Step 1: Select ••• *More*

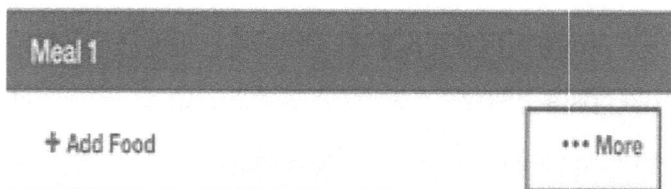

Step 2: Select Turn On Smart Copy

Turn On Smart Copy

Quick Add

Step 3: Swipe right to add

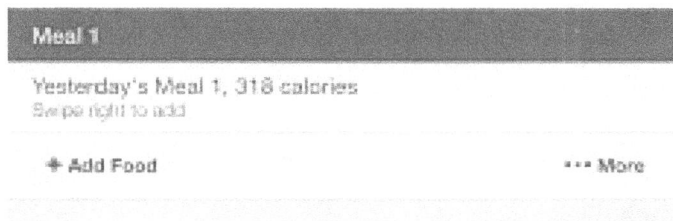

Meal 1

Yesterday's Meal 1, 318 calories
Swipe right to add

+ Add Food   **••• More**

It's as simple as that. You can enable, or disable, this feature for any meal you'd like. Depending on your real situation, you might need to adjust what gets copied. Sometimes you might want to add or remove a particular food that gets copied from the day before. You're able to approve what gets copied and what doesn't.

Meal Plans: The Easiest Way to Use MFP

Meal plans require a little bit of initial work to set up. But once you've got one, it's done, and it's like putting yourself on fat burning auto-pilot mode.

Consider it a better approach than having to ask yourself "Okay consistently... what am I going to eat today?" every few hours of every day. Take the time to create a meal plan and liberate yourself from such decisions.

Take a look at a meal plan I created for myself:

Meal 1:

- Chicken breast (~8-9 oz. uncooked weight)
- Red potatoes (~ 15-16 oz.)
- 2 whole eggs
- 85 grams of broccoli (weighed frozen)
- Light Butter (14 grams)
- Dark Chocolate (1-2 Squares)

Meal 2:

- Chicken Breast (~8-9 oz. uncooked weight)
- Lentil Beans (1 cup)
- Brown Rice (1 cup)
- 1 egg
- 85 grams of broccoli (weighed frozen)
- Light Butter (7 grams)

Meal 3:

- Low Fat Cottage Cheese (1/2 cup)

- Whey Protein (1 scoop)

- Peanut Butter (4 grams)

- Quaker Oats (10 grams)

- Banana (40 grams sliced)

- Stevia Packet

- Walden Farm Zero Calorie Chocolate Syrup

As you can see, I only eat three meals a day and skip breakfast. This is an intermittent fasting example of meal planning, but a meal plan nonetheless. By the way, IIFYM and Intermittent fasting complement each other handsomely, but that a topic for a future book.

The great thing about meal plans is that you can tailor them to your needs. Whether that's three, four, five, or six meals a day! Your pick of foods is up for grabs as long as you hit your daily macros. Be strategic about the foods you pick. Make sure to include nutritiously dense foods in each of your meals to ensure satiety. You can fit treats into your daily macro limit, be aware that you'll most likely not feel full if they're massively spread throughout your meal plan. I recommend having your daily treat alongside one of your meals.

An easy way to a create a meal plan is to brainstorm the foods you like to eat and distribute them amongst the number of meals you'd like to eat every day. You can use grocery items you already have at home and cross-check the nutritional values (macros). Simply scan or search foods in MFP and create a meal plan that fits your macros. Creating a meal plan takes time, so set aside some time to complete this task. I usually start this process by writing down my plan and then transferring the final meal plan into a nice spreadsheet.

Eating Out (Nutrition Info. Available)

Just because you set a fitness goal to improve your health and lifestyle doesn't mean you have to eliminate eating out. Such a tradeoff would be absurd. On days, I know I'm going out to eat, I like to plan.

MFP has an impressive feature called, *Create a New Food* under *My Recipes & Foods* in the main menu.

You can take advantage of using this feature by doing some quick Google research on the place you're going to be dining at. The *Create a New Food* feature allows to you input the calories (and macros) you find from your Google research. This natural process involves Googling nutrition information and configuring what you see in your MFP diary.

Unless you want to ask for nutrition information at the restaurant, then I suggest you do some quick research before going out to eat (for simplicity, I'll be using the word *restaurant* to describe traditional restaurants and fast food places alike).

Do you have a restaurant in mind?

Good, take a look at the example below. It's an example of me creating a new meal entry, in MFP, for a Chipotle Mexican Grill meal:

Step 1: Google: *"restaurant" + nutrition*

Google   chipotle nutrition   🎤 🔍

Step 2: Select the nutrition calculator option if available

Nutrition Calculator - Chipotle
https://www.chipotle.com/nutrition-calculator ▾ Chipotle Mexican Grill ▾
Chipotle Mexican Grill, USA, Canada and UK, Burritos, Tacos and more. Food With Integrity.

Note: Some restaurants will only have nutrition facts and not a calculator. This varies from website to website

Step 3: Choose Your Meal

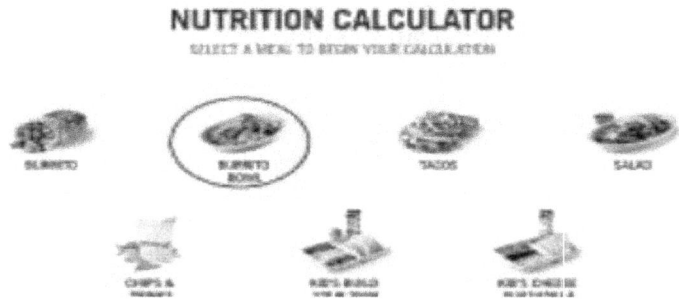

Step 4: Select Your Ingredients

SELECT MEAT OR TOFU

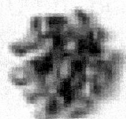 CHICKEN

+ 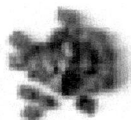 STEAK

+  CARNITAS

Step 5: Check the Nutrition Total: Calories and Macronutrients

TOTALS

SERVING SIZE (OZ)	18.5
CALORIES	650
CALORIES FROM FAT	210
TOTAL FAT (G)	22.5
SATURATED FAT (G)	11
TRANS FAT (G)	0
CHOLESTEROL (MG)	162
SODIUM (MG)	1385
CARBOHYDRATES (G)	61
DIETARY FIBER (G)	15
SUGAR (G)	4
PROTEIN (G)	44

Step 6: Create a New Food in MFP and fill in the details

6a)

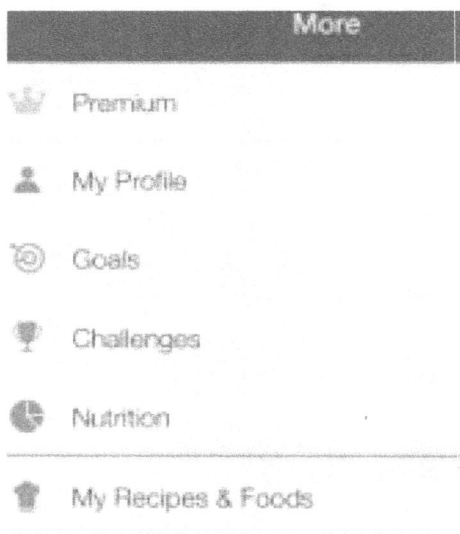

6b)

My Recipes & Foods

Q Search for a food

Foods

6c)

✕	Create Food	→

Brand Name
Optional

Chipotle

Description
Required

Chicken Burrito Bowl w/ Usual

Serving Size
Required

1 Taco Bowl

Servings per container
Required

1

Step 7: Fill in Nutrition Info. (from Step 5)

7a)

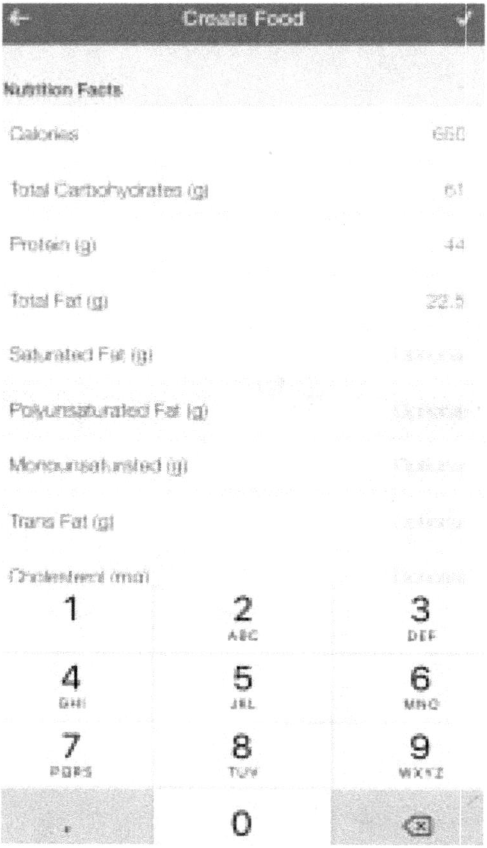

7b)

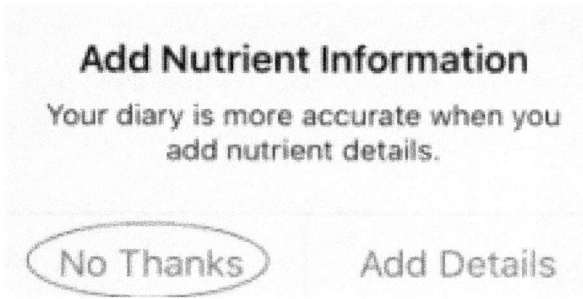

Add Nutrient Information

Your diary is more accurate when you
add nutrient details.

(No Thanks)   Add Details

7c)

←   Lunch

Q Search for a food

Recent   Frequent   (My Foods)

My Foods

Chicken Burrito Bowl w/ Usual
Chipotle, 1 Taco Bowl, 650 calories

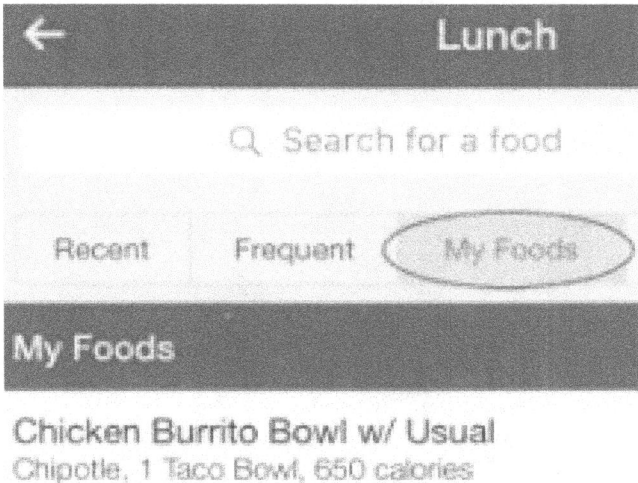

This is great, now I can add a chicken burrito bowl
from Chipotle to any of my meals, whenever I choose
to eat there again. Next time I eat out at Chipotle, I
won't have to redo the process above! You can use
this method for any restaurant meal you enjoy.

Unfortunately, not every restaurant provides easy-to-use online nutrition calculators like Chipotle's website. In most cases, they don't need to. You usually know what you're getting, and expecting, in most cases.

For example, In-N-Out Burger can easily be searched in MFP's database (use Method 1 from Ch. 3). I usually go with a "double-double burger." I search MFP for: "*double-double in n out.*"

This method of eating out looks like this:

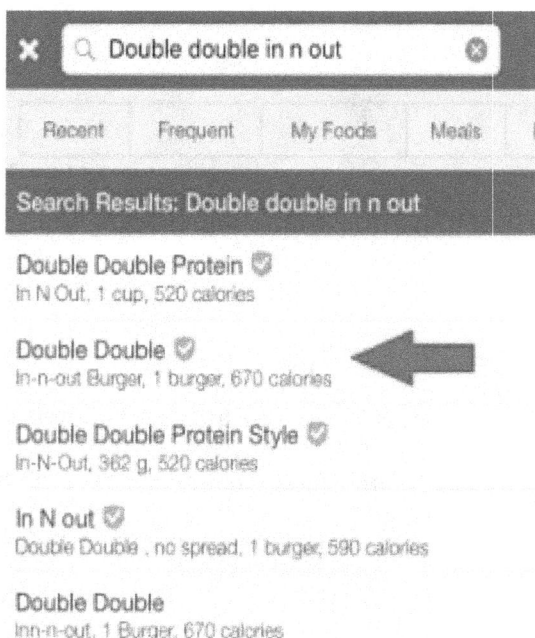

then

Add Food	✓

Double Double (In-n-out Burger) 🛡

Serving Size	1 burger
Number of Servings	1

Nutrition Facts

Calories	670
Fat (g)	41
Saturated (g)	18
Polyunsaturated (g)	0
Monounsaturated (g)	0
Trans (g)	1
Cholesterol (mg)	120
Sodium (mg)	1,440
Potassium (mg)	0
Carbs (g)	39
Fiber (g)	3
Sugars (g)	10
Protein (g)	37

Not too bad right? If you felt like adding fries with that, you know what to do.

Eating Out (Nutrition Info. Unavailable)

There are times when restaurants don't provide nutrition information online or offline. This can be the case if you're in one of those, delicious "hole in the wall" type spots of town. Another occasion could be that you're at a more formal restaurant, eating at a social gathering, like a barbecue, or eating a hot dog at a ball game. Is there a way to log this in? Well, yes and no, we can use a rough estimate approach.

Let's use a traditional restaurant scenario; you've ordered a lean cut of steak and mashed potatoes. You noticed that the steak is 10 ounces according to the menu. The weight of mashed potatoes wasn't given. It's time to bring out MFP and search generic entries for both foods while you wait for the food to be served.

Lunch	595 cal
Steak Steaks, 10 ounce	475
Mashed Potatoes W/ Gravy Generic, 1 cup	120
✚ Add Food	••• More

You can tailor this method to any scenario you encounter. Of course, it's not going to be 100% accurate, but "ballpark" will be good enough for these situations.

There's no reason to skip out on a restaurant meal because nutrition information wasn't available! Just do your best to stay within your caloric deficit, remember that's the key. Some flexible dieters don't log in foods, in such occasions, because it's not worth the hassle, for one, and two, because they know the food they're consuming won't push them over maintenance. Sure their caloric deficit percentage won't be ideal, but they will not gain weight.

If you go overboard, it's not the end of the world. One day of over spillage won't kill you. However, if you make eating out a consistent habit, it might add up to very little visual progress, or worse, set you back for days.

As you can see, there's no silver bullet when it comes to eating out. There are different strategies for different scenarios at best. Being prepared for, at least, one of them makes it easier to gauge your intake and lessens the chances of gaining fat by making you aware of what you're consuming.

Moderation is Key

"If one oversteps the bounds of moderation, the greatest pleasures cease to please." – Epictetus

Everything in moderation. Will you never eat cookies or go out to a fast food joint again? I doubt it; well, I know I couldn't at least. This is why I treat myself to these foods in moderation.

Moderation, in my experience, is having a maintenance day once a week. A day where I eat at equilibrium where I know, I'm not going to be losing or gaining weight. The scale the next morning might rise, but I know it's temporary water weight, glycogen, and most importantly I know it's not weighted from fat.

I usually have maintenance days on Fridays or Saturdays. Eating at maintenance once a week will not hinder your weight loss efforts. I believe they're psychologically necessary. They're almost like reward days if you think about it.

Before I started IIFYM, I used to binge on fast foods. The scenario went like this: full>satisfied>bloated>uncomfortable>" wow why did I do that." And on some occasions, I drank alcohol on the same nights! This is a common combination that leads to fat gain.

It's worth noting that 1 gram of alcohol is equivalent to 7 calories.

When I go out to eat, I stay within my daily macro budget as going out to eat on a maintenance day is just a bonus. What another type of diet allows for this?! Rest assured, as long as it's not a daily habit, fast food is not off limits.

CHAPTER 8: TRACKING YOUR PROGRESS

"Success is nothing more than a few disciplines, practiced every day."

– Jim Rohn

Body composition describes the percentage breakdown of the amount of muscle, body fat, bone and water our bodies are composed of.

You're going to want to be proactive by tracking numbers associated with your weight and waist circumference. You want to understand your body composition as much as possible throughout your fitness journey to always know if you're headed in the right direction.

To make sure you're on the right track, losing fat, not wasting time, and doing so in a healthy manner, measuring your progress is essential. In the words of Lord Kelvin, a physicist & engineer (who determined the correct value of a Kelvin (273°C)), "If you cannot measure it, you cannot control it." Measuring is a part of progressing and should be a weekly habit, and can even be a daily habit.

There are two primary tools, outside of MFP, you're going to use to measure your progress and chances are you have these devices lying around somewhere.

Weight and Pictures

The weight scale is the iconic progress tracker when it comes to weight loss. Although it doesn't provide us with the whole story, on our progress, it's still useful.

Keep in mind that weight fluctuates depending on the time of day you weigh yourself. Throughout your journey, you might weigh yourself one day and seem to have lost a pound, and the next you're back at square one, or sometimes even a pound heavier.

This is normal and is nothing to stress over. Everyone encounters this issue when they're in a caloric deficit, and you're not alone.

Many factors have an impact on weight fluctuations. A few of these factors are water retention, bowel movements, and glycogen storage. To get the most accurate scale reading, we're going to measure by the weekly averages, not days. Weigh yourself at the same time every day. Make sure to do this first thing in the morning, on an empty stomach, as well as, after using the restroom to get the most accurate reading. At the end of every week take the average of your readings and note that it doesn't have to be every day of the week.

MFP can handle tracking your daily weight measurements.

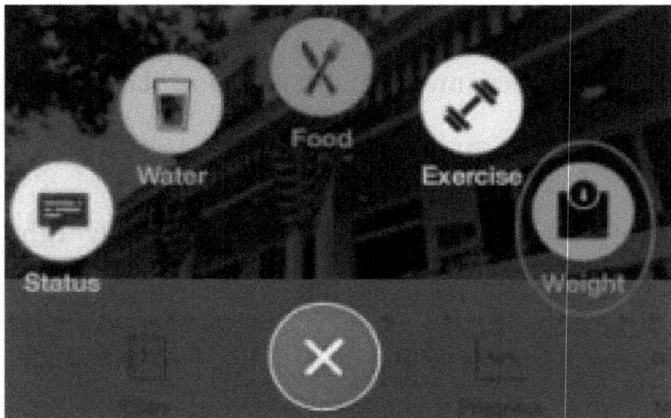

MFP also gives you the option to take photos, which I highly recommend, when you go to record your weight.

Pictures, along with mirror reflection analysis, will help you get a better understanding of how you're progressing. It's also really great to look back at your old photos and compare them with the new you! MFP lets you compare photos side by side, detailing both the date you took the picture and how much you weighed on that day.

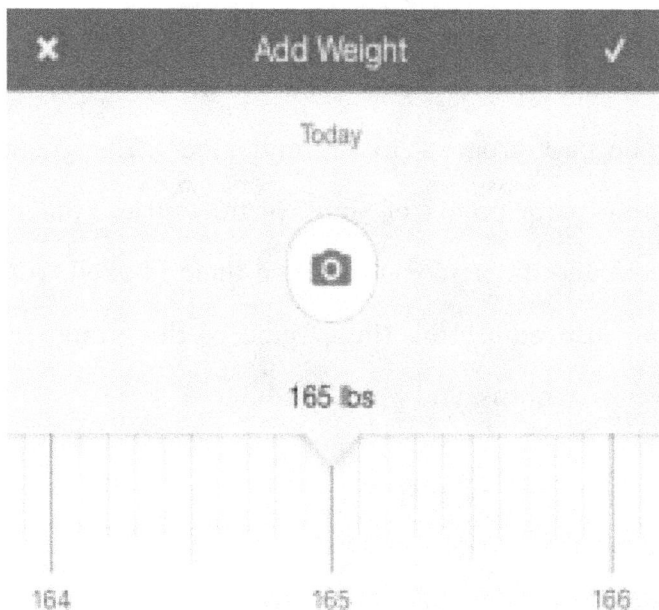

If you'd like to see your progress, at a glance, you can do so by selecting *Progress* in MFP's lower menu.

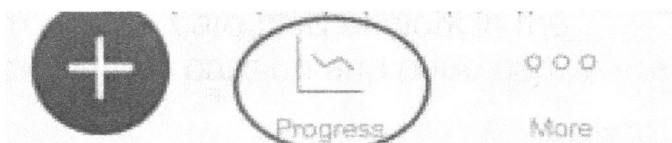

Selecting this will take you to a page where you can view the progress you've made. It allows you to see your past progress in a graph mode. The graph shows data points of your weight entries (the y-axis) and the date you recorded them (x-axis). You can also adjust the time frame of this graph by weeks, months, and years.

This is a handy feature that is much better than keeping a separate journal and having to record every day in my opinion manually. Be consistent, and your graph will end up looking like a beautiful fluctuating mess (you'll see what I mean soon).

Waist

The second method of tracking progress is using a waist tape measure. A tape measure is arguably more revealing than the scale because you can potentially have a smaller weight on the same day the weight on the scale is stagnant. Along with photos, it can be a determining factor, to check, if you've genuinely gained weight or if your body is just retaining water. For those reasons, it's a good idea to measure your waist, just above the belly button, after you weigh in.

To get the most accurate reading, relax and don't suck in your tummy. Breathe as you usually would and get a reading.

MFP will track waist measurements in the same fashion it follows weight.

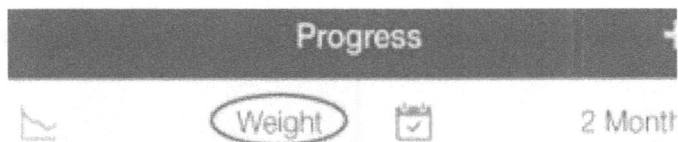

You can change the progress settings by switching "Weight" to "Waist" to record your waist measurement.

Select a Measurement

Weight

Neck

Waist

Hips

BONUS CHAPTER -

FLEXIBLE DIETING RECIPES

The next 3 pages contain a few of my favourite flexible dieting meals. These are easy to fit into your daily macronutrients and very easy to make. I am far from a master chef, so if I can make these - so can you. I eat these meals on a regular basis.

If you enjoy these recipes, be sure to stay tuned for a dedicated recipe and protein smoothie book, which I will be releasing shortly.

Protein Power Pizza

Description:

A delicious miniature protein pizza, this recipe can be altered to suit your personal preference. However, this is a great base to work with.

Ingredients:

Wholemeal Pita Bread

Tomato Paste

Whole Chicken

Baby Spinach

Tomatoes

Mushroom

Cheese (if desired)

Method:

- Spread tomato paste over wholemeal pita bread base

- Cut up chicken and place on pizza (1 whole chicken = 6 pizzas)

- Cover pizza with spinach, mushroom, and tomato

- Place pizzas in over on 200 degrees Celsius (392F) for 20 minutes

Macronutrients

Per pizza

Protein: 50g

Carbohydrates: 45G

Fat: 5G

425 calories

Premium Protein Cheesecake

Description:

Delicious protein cheesecake, this cheesecake can be made in different variations simply by altering the flavour of protein used (change vanilla to chocolate and add some topping) or stick with vanilla and add some berries.

Ingredients:

340 grams (12oz) fat-free cream cheese280 grams (10oz) plain Greek yogurt

2 eggs

2 tbsp. stevia

¼ cup of milk

2 scoops whey protein

1 tsp vanilla extract

Dash of salt

Method:

- Preheat oven to 160 degrees Celsius (320F)

- Soften cream cheese in a large mixing bowl

- Add eggs and stevia, proceed to mix

- Add the remaining ingredients

- Mix all ingredients for 3 minutes

- Pour mixture into baking pan lined with parchment paper

- Bake at 160 degrees Celsius (320F) for 20 minutes then adjust to 90 degrees Celsius (194F) for an hour

- Place in fridge for 5 hours to cool

- Serve with toppings if desired

Macronutrients

per 225 grams (8oz) slice

40g protein

15g carbohydrates

2g fat

238 calories

Mad Monkey Protein Smoothie

Description:

A thick and delicious chocolate smoothie that packs a punch! Great for increasing your energy level before a workout.

Ingredients:

2 scoops chocolate whey protein

100ml skim milk

1 banana

1 tbsp. peanut butter

1 tbsp. coffee

1 cup ice

Method:

- Place all ingredients in a blender or magic bullet and blend for ~20 seconds

- Enjoy!

Macronutrients:

55g protein

32g carbohydrates

15g fat

401 calories

CONCLUSION

Dieting is something we all talk about. People often search for the perfect diet, following each new fad as it appears, hoping that this will be the one that will allow us to make progress. Unfortunately, there is much more chance of failure with each 'fasting' or 'caveman diet' that we try... not necessarily because they don't work, but because they are not something which we can follow over a prolonged period. Any diet that leaves you feeling deprived is almost certainly bound for failure, as is one that goes you bored with the foods that you are allowed to eat. The ONLY way to successfully make progress towards your goals is to change the way you eat.

Flexible dieting will allow you to incorporate the foods you love into your diet in moderation and still make weight loss progress (or lean muscle gains, depending on your goal). There will no longer be the need to stress about what you can eat when you go out socially as certain foods are no longer labeled as 'bad' or 'fattening.' Now that you know how to calculate and track your daily intake, you can look forward to your next meal instead of dreading the thought of having to consume tasteless boiled vegetables.

For me, flexible dieting is the key to living a balanced, healthy lifestyle in a body I am proud to own. Setting goals and achieving them with the help of flexible dieting creates new found confidence in the individual which, in turn, motivates you to stay true to the path of the ongoing journey – it is the flow of positive, constant progression. You're either spiralling up or spiralling up.

I hope you enjoyed reading this book as much as I enjoyed creating it for you. I would like to wish you the best of luck with your flexible dieting, so go out there and achieve your goals!

FINAL WORDS

Thank you again for purchasing this book!

I really hope this book is able to help you.

The next step is for you to **join our email newsletter** to receive updates on any upcoming new book releases or promotions. You can sign-up for free and as a bonus, you will also receive our "*7 Fitness Mistakes You Don't Know You're Making*" book! This bonus book breaks down many of the most common fitness mistakes and will demystify many of the complexities and science of getting into shape. Having all this fitness knowledge and science organized into an actionable step-by-step book will help you get started in the right direction in your fitness journey! To join our free email newsletter and grab your free book, please visit the link and signup: **www.hmwpublishing.com/gift**

Finally, if you enjoyed this book, then I would like to ask you for a favour, would you be kind enough to leave a review for this book? It would be greatly appreciated!

Thank you and good luck in your journey!

Intermittent Fasting

The Ultimate Beginner's Guide To The Intermittent Fasting Diet Lifestyle - Delay, Don't Deny Food - Finally Lose Weight, Burn Fat, Live A Healthier & More Productive Life

By Simone Jacobs

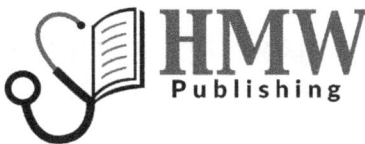

HMW
Publishing

For more great books visit:

HMWPublishing.com

Table of Contents

3

Introduction

Do you have a weight loss problem? Do you continuously watch out for answers in the market hoping for a quick and efficient solution to your problem? If you do, then this book is entirely right for you!

Everyone seems to be in a rush searching for ways to weight loss nowadays. A myriad of offers covering dieting, health and food supplements, physical fitness programs, and various training workshops are flooding the entire health and fitness market. All these entail costs and effort on your part and mostly turn out to be not as effective as these marketers promised in their glamorous ads.

However, there's an ongoing solution that many are resorting to nowadays. Although it is not exempted from cynic opinions, it is a lot better than those options being offered in the market. For one, it does not require your extra effort to do it, and it does not hit your pocket like it does when you prepare for a new set of diet or enrol in a physical fitness program.

The popularity of intermittent fasting is gaining momentum in the market today when people are getting tired of numerous diets that sound easy to do at the first attempt but usually do not work well in the long run.

This book, *"Intermittent Fasting: 7 Beginner's Intermittent Fasting Methods for Women & Men-Weight loss and Build Lean Muscle Hacks"* is designed to provide you with an efficient alternative solution to your problem regarding weight.

This book will further enlighten you about the fundamentals of Intermittent Fasting and how it proves to be the coolest, quickest, and easiest way to lose weight while building lean muscles for both men and women. Grab a copy of this book before it's gone and start dropping pounds in fewer days!

Also, before you get started, I recommend you joining our email newsletter to receive updates on any upcoming new book releases or promotions. You can sign-up for free, and as a bonus, you will receive a free gift. Our *"Health & Fitness Mistakes You Don't Know You're Making"* book! This book has been written to demystify, expose the top do's and don'ts and to finally equip you with the information you need to get in the best shape of your life. Due to the overwhelming amount of mis-information and lies told by magazines and self-proclaimed "gurus", it's becoming harder and harder to get reliable information to get in shape. As opposed to having to go through dozens of biased, unreliable and un-trustworthy sources to get your health & fitness information. Everything you need to help you has been broken down in this book for you to easily follow and to immediately get results to achieve your desired fitness goals in the shortest amount of time.

Once again, to join our free email newsletter and to receive a free copy of this valuable book, please visit the link and signup now: www.hmwpublishing.com/gift

Chapter 1: Lose Weight and Build Muscle on a Time-Tested, Ancient Healing Tradition

The demands and responsibilities of life often lead to various health problems, especially when you are too distracted and you overlook the importance and the practice of a healthy lifestyle and eating habit. More often than not, you do notice the slow changes happening to your body, but you are too busy to do anything about it. The only time you will ever really decide to do something about your concern is when you are already getting sick to the point that you cannot work efficiently.

So your search for solutions begins, but which diet, training, and health fitness program REALLY works? There are tons and tons of them out there. The answer is simple. Teach your body to heal itself and to lose weight by learning when to eat and when to stop eating.

GEAR YOUR BODY, MIND, AND SPIRIT TOWARDS HEALING AND WEIGHT LOSS

Learning when to eat and when to stop eating is a practice called Intermittent Fasting (IF). This concept is nothing new. It's a method used by many people all over the world since time immemorial. Humans go through long periods without eating for most of our history for various religious reasons and when the food source is scarce. In fact, when we sleep, we inadvertently fast.

We fast when we sleep? Yes, indeed! If you typically eat your dinner by 8 pm and have your breakfast at 8 am the morning you wake up, you are fasting for 12 hours and eating for 12 hours. We call this fasting method as a 12/12 fast. Isn't that great news? You can fast while sleeping! I mean it's no effort at all if you choose to practice this method.

But fasting is not exclusive to humans, even animals fast when they are ill or stressed, and sometimes when they feel slightly uneasy. Fasting is a natural tendency for every organism, whether animal or human, to conserve energy during critical times and to seek balance and to rest.

A Brief Glance at the History of Fasting

Hippocrates, Galen, Socrates, Plato, and Aristotle, as well as early great healers, thinkers, and other philosophers all praised the benefits of fasting for healing and health therapy. Paracelsus, one of the three fathers of Western medicine said, "Fasting is the greatest remedy--the physician within."

Early spiritual and religious groups fast as part of their rites and ceremonies, especially during the fall and spring equinoxes. Almost every dominant religion observe fasting for various spiritual benefits.

North and South American Indian traditions, Hinduism, Buddhism, Islam, Gnosticism, Judaism, and Christianity use one form of fasting or another for sacrifice or mourning, penance, spiritual vision, or purification.

Yogic practices, including fasting, date as far back as back as thousands of years. Paramahansa Yogananda, a famous yogi and guru said, "Fasting is a natural method of healing." Likewise, Ayurveda, ancient healing practice, includes fasting as part of its therapy.

However, scientific medicine became dominant and developed better drugs. Fasting and other Naturopathic ways of healing fell off the stage. Recently, many people searching for health solutions return to the old ways.

Modern-Day Fasting

The time-tested, ancient healing tradition of intermittent fasting is back in the spotlight and gaining popularity among many people today. Between 1895-1985, Herbert Shelton, a physician, followed and supervised the fasts of over 40,000 people. During the century and concluded that fasting is a radical and fundamental process that is older than any practice of healing the body, an instinctive method when an organism is sick.

Even though IF is a practice that is as old as the human race itself, modern science and recent studies now reveal that knowing when and eat and when to stop eating creates significant positive changes in the body, resetting the entire system that increases its ability to function at high levels both mentally and physically. Indeed, many research supports the health benefits of IF.

Food abstinence keeps the mind and memory sharp, reduces the risk of various diseases, and keeps the body cells healthy. A study titled, "The Scientific Evidence Surrounding Intermittent Fasting" conducted by Amber Simmons, Ph.D., pointed out that IF together with caloric restriction, is an effective method to promote weight loss in obese and overweight individuals.

Fasting is not Starving

When people hear the word fasting, they often think of it as synonymous to starving. This misconception can often lead people astray and choose other never-been-heard, exotic, and sometimes complicated, diet method.

Starving is when you don't know when your next meal will come. On the other hand, fasting is a practice where you strategically plan periods of when to 'eat' and 'stop eating.' In fact, the word breakfast is the meal you eat to break the fast that you do every day while you are sleeping.

Moreover, it is not the fasting but the caloric restriction that comes with limiting what you eat that produces the health benefits. For example, if you eat at 6 am in the morning and refrain from eating anything within the next 9 hours, then you are actually restricting your calorie without counting, given that you only eat the right amount of food and do not eat double servings of your meal at breakfast. The key to IF is 'discipline,' not starvation.

Teach Your Body to Burn Glucose and Fat

Intermittent Fasting is not a diet per se, but a method in which you teach your body to compartmentalize into "eating" and "fasting" periods. How does learning when to eat and when not to eat help a person lose weight?

Recalibrating a System Dependent on Food

The body metabolizes fat and glucose from the food you eat as its primary source of energy. Carbohydrates are the primary source of glucose. When you eat carb-rich diet, they are broken down into the simpler form called glucose. This substance circulates freely in the bloodstream into every cell of your body as the energy source. When you eat, you supply your body with enough glucose to sustain your body with enough energy to run for 3-4 hours.

Excess glucose goes to the liver and muscles for storage and becomes the body's secondary source of energy. When the cells run out of free circulating blood glucose, the body will break down and metabolize the stored glycogen and transforms it into glucose. Glycogen is the reason you do not have to eat every 15 to 20 minutes. In fact, glycogen stores in your body can sustain you for 6 up to 24 hours after your last meal.

The problem begins when you consume excessive amounts of carbohydrates. Your body runs out of storage capacity for glycogen, so the liver converts it into adipose tissue, triglycerides, or fat for long-term storage. And because you continuously supply the body with energy by eating 3 meals and 2 to 3 snacks in between, the cells consistently have an excess supply of glucose, which is converted into more glycogen in the liver and fat in the body.

Do you see the picture clearer now? Most of us consume more energy than our body can utilize, so the system stores them as glycogen and body fat. We also tend to eat when we feel slightly hungry, so we do not give our cells the chance to use these stored fuels. Thus, we end up adding more and more stored glycogen and adipose tissue into our system, which leads to various health problems, including diabetes, overweight, and other related illnesses linked to high-sugar and high-fat content in the body.

Moreover, when we eat continuously, your body is used to the constant supply of free-circulating glucose, which could lead to insulin resistance. It is a condition where the body is repeatedly with high levels of sugar and insulin in the blood until your system no longer produces sufficient insulin to metabolize glucose or become resistant to its effect.

Make Your Body into a Sugar-and-Fat-Burning Machine

The simple principle behind intermittent fasting is "discipline." **Not feeding or eating for periods gives the body a chance to burn off excess and stored glucose and fat. Practicing IF recalibrates your body from a system that is dependent on food into a sugar-and-fat-burning machine.**

The human body is a fantastic mechanism with a developed system that allows it to deal with periods of low food source. It undergoes the 5 sequent process or stages below to sustain the need for energy.

Feeding

Eating food raises the insulin levels of the body, allowing the tissues of the body to utilize the glucose as energy. During this stage, the liver stores it any excess as glycogen within itself. When the storage space of glycogen in the liver is full, the organ transforms the surplus it into triglyceride or fat for extended storage.

Glycogen Breakdown

Within 6 to 24 hours after your meal, the insulin level will start to fall. During this period, the body will begin metabolizing the stored glycogen as energy and this secondary source of glucose in the liver can sustain the body for about 24 hours.

Gluconeogenesis

After roughly 24 hours up to 2 days without a ready source of glucose, the body utilizes amino acids, the simple form of protein, to manufacture new glucose during the process called "gluconeogenesis." In a non-diabetic person, the glucose levels will fall but stay within the normal range.

Ketosis

After 2 to 3 days without food, the low insulin levels in the body stimulates the breakdown of triglycerides or stored fat for energy during the process called lipolysis. The body metabolizes the stored fat into 3-fatty acid chains and glycerol backbone. The body uses the glycerol for gluconeogenesis or manufacturing of new glucose. The body tissues can readily utilize the 3-fatty acid chains as energy.

However, the brain cannot, so the body metabolizes the 3-fatty acid chains into ketone bodies or energy that can pass in the blood-brain barrier as the brain's fuel source, which is mainly in the forms of acetoacetate and beta-hydroxybutyrate, to sustain the brain's energy needs.

Four days after the body's last meal, 75 percent of the energy used by your mind is from ketones, and the amount increases over 70 times during the fasting period.

On the 5th day, fasting stimulates the production of growth hormone to help the body maintain lean tissue and muscle mass. During this period, the metabolic system utilizes ketones and fatty acids entirely as the source of energy. The level of adrenaline (norepinephrine) also increases to adapt to the change, giving the body more fuel.

Of course, you will not be depriving yourself of food nor be starving during intermittent fasting. As mentioned, IF practice focuses on scheduling when to eat and when not to feed, which gradually teaches the body to utilize excess and stored sugar and fat as energy instead of relying on food. This traditional method opens the gates to better health, weight loss, and building of muscle mass and lean tissue.

Fasting is the Easiest Way to be Healthy

The best thing about intermittent fasting is you can incorporate it into any healthy and balanced diet. When diet is particularly hard to follow, you have the option to stop worrying about what to eat at the very least. It is also convenient when you do not have to prepare meals for a period. Plus, you can save on some amount of money, too. But that's not the real reason why most people love intermittent fasting. There is more to the practicality IF practice offers.

Some people developed the habit of not eating healthy food choices and unhealthy feeding patterns throughout their lifetime, including eating in between meals, choosing fast and junk foods over a well-balanced diet, or just routinely giving in to constant food cravings when they feel hungry. All these constitute an unhealthy lifestyle, which can eventually lead to serious health problems.

Going on a diet and doing a fasting practice both leads to weight loss; hence, people aiming to shed their excess fat face a predicament when choosing which method to adapt to a healthier lifestyle.

According to Dr. Michael Eades, co-author of the famous book, "Protein Power," it is always easy to contemplate on a diet, but it is often harder to execute. Contrary to an eating program, intermittent fasting is just the opposite, it appears to be too hard to contemplate, but once you perform, you find it is not that hard at all.

Going on a diet is always easier during the first few days, but the longer you stay on it, you find it less and less appealing. The reason why most diets do not work out in the long run. Only a few people manage to integrate one form of eating into their lifestyle.

Thinking of fasting would always send you to believe you can't survive a day without eating, especially for those who badly need to fast. However, you will find it easier to do when you start doing it. Turning it into a habit and making it a part of your lifestyle is easier done than just contemplating on it. It's hard to overcome the idea of not eating, but once you go over the hurdle, intermittent fasting is, in fact, easier to do than following a diet.

Intermittent fasting acts as a reset button. It does not regulate nor does not tell you what kind of food you should eat and not consume. Instead, it determines the best time when you should have a proper, healthy, and well-balanced meal. It's an eating pattern that you integrate into your lifestyle to recalibrate your body and improve your health.

Key Takeaways:

- Fasting is a time-tested, ancient healing tradition that can help you lose weight and build muscles.

- The practice of scheduling your feeding time gears your body, mind, and spirit towards various health benefits.

- The key of intermittent fasting is discipline, not starving. It is simply planning when to eat and when not to eat.

- Fasting with caloric restriction recalibrates your body from a sugar-fueled system into a fat-burning machine.

- It resets the button, giving your body the chance to relax and direct energy for healing, weight loss, and muscle building.

Chapter 2: The Virtues of Intermittent Fasting

Before you start fasting, you need to understand what hormonal adaptation your body will undergo concerning fat loss, so you do not immediately plunge into it just to stop before it even starts working on your body.

For starters, let's review the "fed state" and the "fasted state" of the human body. A human body is in a fed state when it is taking in and digesting food. Generally, the feeding starts at the time you start eating the food, and this will last for 3-5 hours while your digestive system is working on it.

While in the fed state, your body cannot burn fat efficiently because of the high level of insulin in the body that enables the sugar to be utilized by the cells as energy.

However, after the digestion process, your body will soon be in the post-absorptive state, which means that your body is no longer working on processing a meal. This period will last from 8 to 12 hours after your last meal, and during this period, your body starts to gain entry to the fasted state. It is during this time that your body begins to burn fat, and your insulin level will begin to lower.

Take note that your body only enters the fasted state 12 hours after your last meal, and since most of us eat 3-6 meals a day, it is rare that your body is getting into this condition; hence, you are depriving your body of experiencing the fat-burning state.

The reason why those who are practicing IF were able to lose fat even without changing the kind and the quantity of food they are eating or how often they have their exercise. Intermittent fasting allows your body to undergo the fat-burning process that you rarely experience when you have your regular eating schedule.

Intermittent fasting maximizes the glycogen and fat-burning mechanism of the body. During the "fasting state," your system undergoes various hormonal adaptations that lead to weight loss and muscle gain.

Decrease Insulin Levels

All food raises the insulin levels in the body. Therefore, the most consistent, efficient, and effective strategy for lowering it is to avoid foods. If you are a non-diabetic person, your blood glucose levels remain normal as your body starts to switch into fat burning. This adaptation is evident in as short as 24-36 hours of fasting. The longer you fast, the longer the duration of reduced insulin and the decrease is more significant.

According to a study titled, "Alternate-day fasting in nonobese subjects: effects on body weight, body composition, and energy metabolism," fasting every other day is an effective method to reduce insulin levels without affecting the normal glucose levels of the body.

Fasting decreases insulin level by 20-31 percent and lowers your blood sugar by 3-6% once your body utilizes stored fat starts as fuel in place of carbohydrates, thus, likewise reducing the risk for Type 2 diabetes.

Boost Weight Loss

Another reason why intermittent fasting is popular these days is that scientific studies prove it is a powerful technique for weight loss. We love to eat food rich in carbohydrates and fats, and then we panic once we see our weight measurement rise.

With an IF practice, you can choose between eating fewer meals or entirely not consume any food for a few days. This process is sure to reduce the overall calorie intake, as well as normalize the hormonal change that inhibits fat burning as it triggers the release of norepinephrine (noradrenaline).

Through short-term fasting, you can increase your metabolic rate up to 14 percent. Intermittent fasting likewise results in weight loss by changing your caloric equation, e.g., taking in fewer calories and burning more of it.

The same study that showed the effects of alternate-day fasting in reducing insulin levels further revealed after 22 days, the 16 people who ate every other day lost 2.5 percent of their body weight.

The study further showed that their hunger increased during the first fasting day and remained high. There was no significant change in their resting metabolic rate (RMR) and respiratory quotient (RQ) from day 1 to day 21, but on the 22nd day, their RQ decreased, which resulted in a significant increase in fat oxidation or loss in their bodies up to 15 grams and more.

However, since hunger on fasting days did not decrease, the authors of the research suggested that eating a small meal during fasting days make this approach more acceptable. Nevertheless, the study corroborated that fasting is an efficient and fast strategy to lose excess weight.

Burn Belly Fat Faster

Belly fat or what we call the "love handles" are the most dangerous of all the fats stored in your body. The name may sound appealing, but love handles are very sinister. They are hazardous visceral fats that tend to build around the internal organs and later lead to severe illnesses.

However, a study revealed that undergoing intermittent fasting not only reduce body weight; it also decreases waist circumference by 4 to 7 percent.

Stimulate the Production of Growth Hormone

Growth hormone (HG) or somatotropin or human growth hormone (HGH or hGH) stimulates cell reproduction and regeneration and growth, thus, is very vital to human development. It is a natural hormone produced by the pituitary gland, and the majority of the secretion occurs during sleep. As you age the level of HG production declines and it can lead to decreased lean muscle mass, lack of energy, and increase in body fat.

The relationship between human growth hormone and insulin is a complicated one. HGH is the antagonist of the latter and vice versa. When you have insulin resistance, your body continually has high amounts of insulin to balance the high volume of glucose in your body, which decreases the production of GH.

On the other hand, insulin resistance may be the result of HGH deficiency. When your body produces high levels of growth hormone, it competes with the same receptor sites as insulin and instead of metabolizing glucose as the source of energy, the cells burn fat instead. Insulin production decreases and the system cannot adequately stabilize the high amount of sugar in the body. Moreover, people with decreased HGH tend to have excessive body fat content. They also have reduced exercise tolerance and muscle strength.

The fed state inhibits HGH secretion since the body raises the levels of insulin to metabolize the glucose from your food as the source of energy when you eat. Fasting for as little as 5 days increases the secretion of human growth hormone by up to 2 times. When you are fasting, you are decreasing the supply of glucose in the body, which reduces the production of insulin. When the amount of insulin in the body is low, the amount of GHG increases to adapt to the change, burning fat for the energy it needs and losing weight in the process.

Increase growth hormone levels in the body raise the amounts of circulating insulin-like growth factor I (IGF-I), which also regulate growth. The increase of both GHG and IGF-I results in the growth of muscle mass, as well as increase muscle strength.

Increase Adrenaline Levels

Our body is equipped with a survival mechanism that triggers it to go into a survival mode when you are hungry or tired. So when it becomes desperate, the body enhances this instinct so you can have more energy to move and hunt for food.

When you are fasting, your body experiences mild stress that boosts adrenaline production. It is similar to how your body responses when you are exercising or when a dog chases you on the way home. Your natural fight-or-flight hormone kicks in to ensure your safety or survival during dangerous occurrences. Generally, the higher the stress, the higher the adrenaline secretion occurs.

Intermittent fasting is a great way to put your body under stress without actually putting yourself in danger. As your cells start to utilize fat as the source of energy, it signals the body that you need to forage – a primitive instinct that allows early humans to hunt and search for food during times source is scarce, ensuring survival.

Practicing IF naturally stimulates adrenaline secretion, which unlocks and utilizes stored energy – muscle glycogen and fat. Simply put, adrenaline promotes the release of stored glucose from its locations in the body, increasing metabolism even during rested state. Moreover, increased adrenaline levels boost concentration, focus, and energy.

Regulates Functions of Cells, Hormones, and Genes

Once you are in the fasted state, your body initiates repair of cells and regulates your hormone levels to have your body fat working. Here are examples of some changes that occur while you are fasting.

Repair Cells

The body induces some cellular repair, like removing toxins and wastes from your body, in a process known as autophagy, which involves breaking down dysfunctional proteins that have built-up inside the cells over time. Increased autophagy can provide your body protection against several diseases, including cancer and Alzheimer's disease.

Alters Gene Expression

A study titled "The effects of fasting on the physiological status and gene expression; an overview" revealed that calorie restriction through reduction of food or eliminating food and caloric beverages for a period changes various signaling pathways and the expression of different genes, leading to longer lifespan and high immunity against diseases.

Moreover, another study revealed that alternate day fasting increased the expression or SIRT1, a gene linked to longevity. Also, another study showed that gene expression in adipogenesis in mice was also altered, leading to faster regulation of reserved triacylglycerol into fuel.

Relieve Inflammation

Researchers disclosed through studies that intermittent fasting shows a significant reduction in inflammation, which is a crucial determinant for many chronic illnesses. A study titled "Ghrelin gene products in acute and chronic inflammation" showed that reducing food and caloric intake increases the production of ghrelin or the hunger hormone, which suppress chronic and acute inflammation, as well as autoimmunity. Low levels of fat tissue also favor the production of anti-inflammatory proteins.

Develop Strong Heart

Intermittent fasting reduces risk factors for heart diseases, including inflammatory markers, blood triglycerides, LDL cholesterol, blood sugar and insulin resistance. A study titled, "Fasting-induced changes in the expression of genes controlling substrate metabolism in the rat heart" revealed that during IF the heart adapts to the changes in glucose and fatty acid metabolism by altering the cardiac energy production at the level of gene expression. This effect reduces fatty acids in the heart.

Moreover, "Intermittent fasting: the next big weight loss fad" stated that IF produce similar effects as intense exercise, heart rate variability while reducing resting heart rate and blood pressure.

Anti-Aging

When tested in rats, intermittent fasting had extended the animal's lifespan by about 83 percent longer. "Intermittent fasting: the next big weight loss fad" revealed that reducing calorie intake in most animals increased lifespan by up to 30 percent. "Dietary restriction in cerebral bioenergetics and redox state" showed that IF delays the appearance of aging markers.

Moreover, "Caloric restriction (CF) and intermittent fasting: Two potential diets for successful brain aging" pointed out that CF and IF practice affects oxygen radical and energy metabolism, as well as systemic cellular stress response, in a manner that protects that neurons against environmental and genetic factors related to aging.

Improve Your Focus and Mental Clarity

As mentioned earlier, fasting stimulates adrenaline secretion that help boosts concentration, focus, and energy. In Chapter 1: Diet on a Time-Tested,

Ancient Healing, we also tackled ketones and how fasting the assists the body achieve ketosis, making it a fat-burning machine. During ketosis, the liver breaks down fatty acids into ketones as energy.

Ketones are more efficient fuel for the brain than glucose. When your body burns fuel, either ketones or glucose, it converts it into adenosine triphosphate (ATP), the substance that your cells use as energy. Ketones help produce and increase ATP production better than glucose, creating more energy for the body and the brain to use, thus improving mental performance.

Moreover, other research shows that ketones can process gamma-Aminobutyric acid (GABA) more efficiently. GABA is a molecule that reduces brain stimulation.

When you are not fasting, the body utilizes glucose as its primary source of energy and the brain uses glutamic acid and glutamate for fuel, molecules that stimulate brain function. However, when the brain utilizes the glutamic acid and glutamate as fuel, there is little of the two molecules left to process GABA. Your mind starts to over process without a way to reduce the stimulation, your brain neurons are overstimulated and work excessively, which lead to brain fog or what is known as the inability to recall information or focus on a task. Simply put, too much glutamate means too much brain excitement, which results in brain neurotoxicity, which in some cases lead to seizures, as well as various neurological disorders, such as dementia, amyotrophic lateral sclerosis (ALS), migraines, bipolar disorder, and even depression.

When you are fasting, you give the brain another source of energy, which provides the brain with sufficient supplies of glutamic acid and glutamate for processing GABA. This process helps balance and reduces the excess firing of neurons, leading to better mental focus. Moreover, studies show that increased production of GABA reduces anxiety and stress, which also helps improve mental clarity.

Release Energy for Healing

Have you ever worked for more than 8 to 10 hours a day with a massive project, especially when the boss asks you to do something beyond your pay grade or job title? Then you have a precise idea how your body feels when it has to process the food you eat 24 hours a day, 7 days a week.

You put your body under duress. Similar to the way you cope with a considerable workload, your body will deal. It must cope and make important decisions. It attends to the most urgent and important tasks first, setting aside matters that can wait for another day. The more you stuff yourself with food, the more you put it into overwork, whether it is ready or not to take on a new job. Eventually, it cannot keep up, and you experience various health problems. Just like a mean boss dumping another stack of papers to process when you still have 3 tall piles on your desk.

You can take a vacation when you are feeling weary, under-appreciated, and overworked. Your body on the other hand, rarely gets a break, mainly when you eat almost every hour of the day.

Fasting is giving your body its well-deserved vacation from constant feeding. When you eat, the digestive system utilizes up to 65 percent of the energy. Digestion, along with all the other process it needs for the day takes a lot of energy. At the end of the day, your body does not have enough fuel for other essential tasks.

During intermittent fasting, your body diverts energy towards recuperation and healing. Moreover, when you fast, your body undergoes detoxification, efficiently eliminating metabolic wastes naturally produced by healthy cells, as well as foreign toxins. Your system can also spend more fuel on the cell, tissue, and organ repairs instead of just eliminating the byproducts of eating.

Fasting will allow your body to catch up on the critical tasks that it has put aside. During this period, the system will finally be able to handle all the toxins, cleaning the excess toxins from the tissues, thus, creating a stage or an environment for healing.

Fosters Spiritual Growth

As you continually remove heavy and unhealthy food from your diet and detoxify, your body will feel less dense and become lighter. Shedding all the excess fat during the process also makes you lighter. Moreover, fasting reduces sleep disorders and fatigues, helping you attain inner harmony and balance.

When you are healthier, your focus will shift from the worldly things and physical reality towards the aspects of your life that indeed matter instead of your health problems.

The practice of intermittent fasting also fosters discipline, which sharpens spiritual senses, mainly when you practice it together with meditation. Completing self-imposed tasks strengthens your willpower, thus, teaching you to manage your life better, particularly during stressful situations.

Reasons Why Fasting Works

Aside from people's obsession with excess fat and weight loss, there are other reasons why you need to practice intermittent fasting as often as you can, depending on your state of health. Here are few reasons why.

Relaxing

Once you are fasting, there's nothing much to worry about as you don't need to prepare something for your meal not worry about the kind of meal that will have adverse effects on your health. You can just gulp down a glass of water and start your day. Imagine when you have one meal less in a day or one whole day without the regular meals. One day spent less on preparing food is one more day to pamper yourself with a full relaxation. However, it doesn't mean, however, that when you're fasting, you will look gloomy or ash-fallen.

Most of you will probably be expecting someone less energetic or downfallen when on fasting. However, if you ask those who are into fasting, you will be surprised to know how energetic they seem while at this stage that when they are regularly eating their meal.

Lengthens Life Span

It is common knowledge that restricting calories are one of the ways of prolonging life. Hence, when you are fasting, your body is finding a way of extending your life. When you are on the intermittent diet, your body is activating the calorie restriction in response to lengthening your life. With this, you get the benefit of extended life without really experiencing real starvation. A study about alternate day intermittent fasting in mice done way back in 1945 proves that fasting indeed led to a longer lifespan.

Complement Chemo Therapy

There is this study of cancer patients that disclosed the side effects of chemotherapy. According to the study, patients who undergo fasting before the treatment experience diminished these side effects. Moreover, a study asserts that IF significantly increases the impact of chemotherapy or radiation. Further, research backs up on the alternate-day intermittent fasting, which leads to a conclusion that IF before chemotherapy session results in higher positive result rates and fewer deaths. In a comprehensive analysis of various studies of diseases and fasting, it appears that intermittent fasting does reduce not only the risk of cancer but also has a positive effect on cardiovascular diseases.

Key Takeaways:

- During intermittent fasting, your body undergoes various hormonal adaptations, including decrease insulin levels, stimulate the production of growth hormone, increase adrenaline levels, and regulate cell, hormone, and gene functions.

- The various hormonal changes your body undergoes during fasting helps boost weight loss, burn belly fat faster, repair cells, alter gene expression, relieve inflammation, develop strong heart, lengthens lifespan, and release energy for healing, as well as compliment chemotherapy.

- Aside from the positive physical effects, fasting improves your focus and mental clarity, as well as foster spiritual growth.

Chapter 3: Effectively Adapting to the Healthy Change

During caloric restriction (CR) and intermittent fasting, your body will be undergoing changes that could be 360 degrees different from your usual eating habits and the amount of food you consume every day. It will transition from a glucose-fueled system into a fat-burning machine.

The CR and IF will initiate various processes and adaptations until your body is ultimately transformed into a healthy, efficient system. Among the concerns and effects, you need to prepare for the following. Knowing what you have to deal with during fasting will ensure that you successfully adjust to these health practices.

Electrolyte Deficiency

There are misplaced concerns about CR and IF causing malnutrition. These misconceptions are just not correct. The body contains sufficient amount of stored glycogen and fat as the source of energy.

The primary concern during fasting is micronutrient deficiency. However, studies reveal that even prolonged IF do not cause malnutrition. Potassium levels may slightly decrease. However, even 2 months of continuous practice does not reduce the levels below 3.0 milliEquivalents per liter (mEq/L), even without supplements, which is just slightly below the average level of 3.5-5.0 mEq/L. Two months of continues fasting is more extended than recommended and you would not be doing this method on the IF.

On the other hand, phosphorus, calcium, and magnesium remain stable during fasting, which is presumably due to the large stores of them in the bones - about 90 percent of the body's phosphorus and calcium.

Taking a multi-vitamin supplement during CR and IF provides the body of the recommended daily micronutrient allowance. In fact, a 382-day therapeutic fast with multivitamin showed to have no detrimental effect on health. The only related result was the slight uric acid elevation, which exhibited after the hundredth day of fasting.

Uric Acid Elevation

"A study of the Retention of Uric Acid during Fasting" revealed that a 21-fasting period caused a significant increase of the concentration of uric acid in the blood, which was the result of the decreased elimination uric acid. Reduced urine volume seems to be the leading cause of the build-up, as well as the changes in metabolism and kidney functions the system undergoes during IF. The study further stated that ketosis seems to alter the oxidation and the acid-base equilibrium of the body tissues and blood that result in a uric acid increase.

To prevent and/or remedy this side effect, you must:

- Drink sufficient amount of water to dilute uric acid and help the kidneys excrete it more efficiently.

- Increase the alkalinity of the body by eating more vegetables during the feeding period. You can ass boiled beans and peas into your meals to add alkalinity and fullness taste.

- If you have high uric acid before starting fasting, then going vegan or vegetarian might be a good idea.

- Add 1/2 teaspoon baking soda in a glass of water and drink 3 times a day.

- Reduce meat because they contain high purine.

- Avoid alcoholic drinks. Drink coffee or tea instead.

- Blueberries and cherries help reduce pain due to the formation of uric acid crystals.

After-Fast Weight Gain

Gaining weight after the fasting period is normal. The added weight is mostly water weight gain, and you might acquire some fat. Short-term weight gain happens after you break your fats. Once you start eating again, you will see the added weight on your scale.

Do not worry! This gain is temporary. Stored glycogen in the body is heavily hydrated because they are bound to water. During fasting, you use the stored glycogen for energy, so you lose weight. When you enter the feeding state, you will gain water weight as your body replenishes glycogen stores. Moreover, sodium also retains water, which also adds to water weight gain.

This almost immediate additional weight is not excess fat. It is just your body getting back to normal after fasting. Moreover, restricting your calorie intake during fasting drives your body to increase stored energy or body fat for a future period with reduced calories.

Do not fret! More importantly, do not worry. Your body is still transitioning from a glucose-fueled system into a fat-burning machine. Your body will not adapt to the changes right away. But as you continue your fasting practice, your body will soon efficiently utilize fat as its source of energy and burn them. Here are tips to help your body adapt to a fat-fueled system faster.

- Avoid junk and food, alcohol, and sugar, especially during the first week of fasting. These foods provide the body with glucose that feeds fat deposits during the transition period when the body is driven to increase energy storage.

- Consume low glycemic carbohydrates, such as vegetables, legumes, beans, and whole grains. These foods are digested slower, preventing the surge of blood sugar that the body turns into fat as it seeks to replenish energy stores when you break your fast.

- Consume high-quality protein, such as seeds and nuts, legumes, beans, whole grain, low-fat dairy, fish, and meat. They decrease hunger and reduce the body's dependency on carbs for energy, as well as help promote muscle growth.

- Consume low-calorie-density food, such as whole grains and vegetables. They are high in fiber and low in calories per bite, which reduce the sugar you feed your body.

Lean Muscle Mass Loss

This issue is another crucial concern relating intermittent fasting. Does IF burn muscle? The straight answer is NO. In fact, a study revealed that during fasting, the body does not start burning muscle, it starts conserving it. Moreover, physiologic studies concluded that protein is not 'burnt' for glucose.

When the body achieves the state of ketosis, there is no need to use protein for gluconeogenesis or converting amino acids into glucose because the body metabolizes fatty acids as the source of energy. During normal conditions, the body breaks down 75 grams of protein daily. However, during fasting, this falls to about 15 to 20 grams daily. So IF actually decreases muscle breakdown.

Moreover, intermittent fasting boosts the levels of growth hormone and insulin-like growth factor I that promote muscle growth and increased muscle strength.

If you are worried about the lean muscle mass loss, then provide the body with sufficient sources of fatty acid to burn as energy.

Not Everyone Can Fast

Intermittent Fasting is not for everyone. Like other health programs, there are significant rules and exemptions.

Those Who Shouldn't Fast

If you belong to these types of people, then it is advisable for you not to fast.

- Diabetic and hypoglycemic patients
- Those who are underweight
- Those with low blood pressure
- Those with eating disorder
- Those who are under medications
- Pregnant and breastfeeding women
- Women with amenorrhea and fertility problems
- Women who are trying to get conceived
- Those with cortisol deregulation
- Those suffering from chronic stress

Consult a healthcare professional or your doctor if you are uncertain that you can fast. If you have determined that you cannot practice, you can do a cleansing diet instead to detoxify and gain many, if not all, of the benefits of fasting. Cleansing options often create the same detox effects as IF, eliminating toxins and rebuilding healthy tissue, but in a gradual manner.

Fasting for Women

There is some evidence that shows that fasting is less beneficial to women as it is for their male counterparts. It turns out that women's bodies react differently to IF than men's bodies. Females are more sensitive to the signals of hunger. Additionally, the hormones that regulate vital functions like ovulation are extremely sensitive to energy intake. Some women do just fine with intermittent fasting while others experience problems. Even short-term CR and IF can alter the hormonal pulses in some females, disrupting regular and specific cycles.

Moreover, if not done correctly, caloric restriction and intermittent fasting can cause various hormonal imbalances. When the female body senses that it is hungry, it will increase the production of hunger hormones, ghrelin, and leptin. This reaction is the body's way to protect a potential fetus, even when the woman is not pregnant.

Of course, when you are practicing CR and IF, you will ignore these hunger signals, causing the body to produce more hunger hormones, which can throw everything out of balance.

Although there are no studies conducted in humans, rat experiments revealed that intermittent fasting had some adverse effects on female rats. It developed these female rats into masculine-like, infertile, and emaciated rats while causing them to miss cycles. The ovaries shrunk and the menstrual cycles stopped while they experienced more insomnia than males. Moreover, studies show that CR and IF can aggravate eating disorders like bulimia, anorexia, and binge eating disorder.

So how do women approach caloric restriction and intermittent fasting?

Intermittent Fasting Options for Women

For women, the general guidelines for successful IF are as follows:

- Fasting should not last more than 24 hours for periods.

- Women should fast for about 12 to 16 hours only.

- Avoid fasting on consecutive days during the first 2 to 3 weeks of IF. For instance, if you are doing a 16-hour fast, do it 3 days a week instead of 7 days.

- Drink plenty of fluids during your fast, such as water, herbal tea, and bone broth.

- During fasting days, only do light exercises, such as gentle stretching, jogging, walking, and yoga.

Also, several intermittent fasting methods are suitable for women. Here are the most popular ones that you can try.

Crescendo Method

This method is the best way for women to ease into caloric restriction and intermittent fasting without disrupting hormones or shocking the body. This type does not require a female to fast a week, only for a couple of days spaced throughout the period.

For example, fasting for 12 to 16 hours every Monday, Wednesday, and Friday with an eating window of 8 to 12 hours.

The other 3 IF methods best suited for women are the 16/8 Method or the Leangains method, the Eat-Stop-Eat or 24-Hour Protocol, and the 5:2 Diet, which are all discussed in Chapter 4: Listen to the Needs of Your Body.

Stop intermittent fasting if you experience any of the following. These symptoms often indicate that you are experiencing a hormonal imbalance.

- When menstrual cycle becomes irregular or stops

- Experience problems staying or falling asleep

- Falling hair, acne breakout, and dry skin

- Having a hard time recovering from workouts

- Injuries heal slowly and getting sick more often

- The heart starts to beat irregularly or in a weird-manner

- Having mood swings

- Experiencing decreased tolerance to stress

- Feeling cold

- Digestion significantly slows down

- Less interested in sex

Key Takeaways:

- Changing your eating schedule and habit can cause some concerns, such as electrolyte deficiency, uric acid elevation, after-fast weight gain, and lean muscle loss. However, studies show that you can quickly remedy all these side effects.

- Research shows that fasting does not reduce the amount of electrolyte in the body significantly.

- Taking a multi-vitamin supplement during fasting provides the body of the recommended daily micronutrient allowance.

- Fasting can cause a slight elevation in uric acid, but you can easily prevent this from occurring by drinking plenty of water and increasing your alkalinity by eating more vegetables.

- After-fast weight gain is temporary, and most of it is water weight while you are on your regular feeding periods. As you continue fasting, your body will soon efficiently utilize fat as its source of energy and burn them, and your weight will go down eventually.

- Avoid junk and food, alcohol, and sugar, especially during the first week of fasting. Consume low glycemic carbohydrates, such as vegetables, legumes, beans, and whole grains.

- Intermittent fasting does not burn muscle. In fact, boosts the levels of growth hormone and insulin-like growth factor I that promote muscle growth and increased muscle strength. If you are worried about the lean muscle mass loss, then provide the body with sufficient sources of fatty acid to burn as energy.

- Not everyone can fast.

- Women react differently to fasting than men. For effective intermittent fasting, women need to follow a guideline that will prevent disruption of hormonal balance, which is very sensitive to hunger.

- The best fasting methods for women are the Crescendo Method, the 16/8 Method or the Leangains method, the Eat-Stop-Eat or 24-Hour Protocol, and the 5:2 Diet.

- Women should stop fasting when they experience the symptoms of hormonal imbalance.

Chapter 4: Listen to the Needs of Your Body

Fasting recalibrates your body. Practicing this weight loss method without preparation is a recipe for failure. Knowing what you'll have to deal with and choosing the best fasting method will ensure success.

Buffer Your Weight Loss and Muscle Gain Journey

Slow is the way to go, especially if you are just starting on your diet. Preparation will help your body adjust and adapt to the practice better, and help you experience less or no transition symptoms or keto flu (flu-like symptoms a person experiences as the body changes from burning glucose to fat as the primary source of energy). Planning also lessens or prevents detoxification symptoms; fasting can start a release of too many toxins into the bloodstream at one time.

Start Your Diet with a 1-Day Fruit or Juice Fast

Do this once every week until you no longer experience the detoxification symptoms or your body is ready to transition from a glucose-fueled system to fat-burning machine. An apple fruit fast is easy to begin. Start your IF the night before. Eat a light dinner. Do not overfeed yourself out of fear for the next day. On your fasting day, eat 3-4 apples as your meals and drink at least 2 quarts of water throughout the day. Cut back on caffeinated drinks on your apple fruit fast as well. If you crave for something warm during the period, drink warmed water. The next day, when you break your fast, ease into food slowly and then return to regular eating.

When your body is over the detox symptoms, try the Leangains Method (16:8 Fasting) or do a 1-day water fast. People find it easier to deal with the hunger when they slowly ease into an advanced fasting method than jumping immediately into it since the body gradually adjusts to the prospect of not feeding. You will not get too hungry right away, which is something that is difficult to deal with for some people. Eventually, your system will adjust to the no food period.

When your body has sufficiently adapted to the semi-fasting state, you can start with any of the 7 methods below. Before you proceed with your actual fasting, read them all. Weigh your options. Take an honest look at your life. How much can you sacrifice? An IF practice will create intense detoxifying and cleansing symptoms, as well as ketosis symptoms, which will require more discipline from you. How much discomfort can you take?

Do you want a fasting without a great deal of discipline? That is also very possible. Some professionals suggest avoiding extreme symptoms of detoxification by doing an easy fasting method. You can absolutely take it slower, at a pace most comfortable for you.

#1 - Leangains Method (16:8 Fasting)

Started by Martin Berkhan, Leangains Method is best recommended for dedicated fitness enthusiasts aiming to lose body fats and build muscles.

Under the Leangain method of fasting, you are allowed to eat only within 8 or 10 hours break while you are fasting for 16 hours (for men) and 14 hours (for women). During your fasting period, you are not supposed to consume calories though you are permitted to take calorie-free foods.

It is much easier to start fasting through the night until the next morning - roughly six hours after waking up. However, this needs a close maintenance feeding window else you get it harder to stick to the program while disrupting your hormones normal functioning.

The time and the kind of food that you will be eating during your feeding window largely depend on when you will be working out. On days when you are doing your workout, carbohydrates are more important than fat. However, on your rest days, you must take more fats. It is advisable to be always high on protein consumption, but it must be in proportion to your goal, gender, activity level, and body fat. Regardless of how you spend your activity, the consumption of whole and unprocessed food is preferable in choosing your calorie intake. Nonetheless, if you don't have much time for a proper meal, better grab yourself a protein bar or protein shake instead.

For most people who are into this fasting method, the highlight is the fact that in most days, meal frequency does not really matter. You can always eat anytime you want as long as it is within the eight-hour feeding window. With this, most people prefer breaking it up into three meals as it is easier to stick to it while being programmed to this eating habit.

Nonetheless, even if your eating time is flexible, Leangains fast is very specific with its guidelines regarding the kind of food that you can eat, primarily if you are working out. The rather strict guide on nutrition planning makes the program a little bit tough to adhere.

#2 - Eat Stop Eat (24-Hour Fasting)

This program involves fasting for 1 whole day (24 hours) once or twice a week. While you are fasting, you are allowed to drink calorie-free drinks. After the fasting period, you can go back to regular eating.

This method of fasting reduces overall calorie intake without putting a limit on what you eat and how often you want to eat. It is worthy to note, however, that incorporating regular workouts, including resistance training is the bottom line if your goal is a weight loss of an improved body composition.

Though it is quite hard to contemplate that you will be without food for 24 hours, still there is an excellent side of the Eat Stop Eat Fast since this option is quite flexible. You don't have to follow the rule strictly on your first day of fasting. You can go as long as you can manage and then gradually increase your fasting duration over time to give your body enough time to adjust.

It is advantageous if you start your fasting on the day when you are busy and at a time that doesn't fall on your eating schedule like lunch. Another bonus is that there are no forbidden foods, no restrictions on your diet, and no calorie counting. Even the quantity of your food intake is never an issue here. However, you must know how to moderate your eating like you can eat a slice of the cake but not the whole piece.

The long hours of Eat Stop Eat Fast prove to be challenging to some people, especially for starters. While your body is still adjusting, you can feel some symptoms like fatigue, weakness, headache or dizziness, and cranky. All these will tempt you to put a break to your fasting. However, these symptoms diminish over time while it takes a lot of self-control on your part to overcome all those negative feelings.

#3 - The Warrior Diet (20/4 Diet)

This method, which is inspired by the eating habits of warriors in the olden days, allows you fast for 20 hours every day and then eat one large meal in the evening. It is crucial to eat a quality meal rather than getting a hefty one while on your feeding period. Nonetheless, you are allowed mild consumption during the day like a few servings of raw fruits and veggies, or a few servings of protein shakes if you feel like needing it. Some warrior dieters question this option based on the logic that if you exercise this perk, then it's no longer a real fast.

This method of intermittent fasting is supposed to promote alertness, stimulates fat burning, and boost energy while maximizing the fight or flight reaction of the sympathetic nervous system. The four hours feeding state is aimed towards maximizing the ability of the parasympathetic nervous system to help the body to recuperate. Likewise, it promotes calmness, relaxation, and digestion as it helps the body generate hormones and burn fat in the daytime. Further, the order in which you eat specific food groups also matters. According to this method, you should start with vegetables, fats, and proteins. If you are still not satiated, only then will you take in some carbohydrates.

Many prefer this method of intermittent fasting as this option allows you to eat a few small meals or snacks, which can help you get through your fasting period. Many testified to have gained an increase in energy level and fat loss while on this diet.

It may be better to have a few snacks than going without any food for more than 20 hours. Still, to have strict guidelines of what needs to be eaten and when to eat them proves challenging in the long run. Also, eating one main meal at night as according to the guidelines is not easy, especially for folks who prefer minimal intake in the later part of the day.

#4 – Fat Loss Forever

The Fat Loss Forever method is a hybrid of the three practices – Eat Stop Eat, the Warrior Diet, and the Leangains as you combine them all into one single plan. You are also allowed one cheat day for each week and then follow it up by a 36-hour fast. The remainder of the one-week cycle is then split up between the different fasting methods.

In this method, it is recommended that you save the most extended fast on days when you are at your most active level. The practice allows you to focus on your productivity that on your hunger. Integrated into this intermittent fasting are training programs, free weights, and body weights, which are geared towards helping trainees maximize fat loss efficiently.

Founders of this program, John Romaniello, and Dan Go believe that everyone is practically fasting every day and these are times when we aren't eating anything and on an irregular schedule which is why we can't reap the benefit of intermittent fasting. Under the Fat Loss Forever method, there is a seven-day schedule for fasting, which helps your body get used to a structured timetable. It also includes a full-fledged cheat day, which makes the program preferable to many.

Conversely, you will have a hard time handling the cheat days because the plan is too specific and the schedule of fasting or feeding varies from day to day making it confusing to follow. If you are the type who would find it hard to quickly switch from indulging in moderation and then turning it off when it's time to change to fasting, then this program may not work well with you.

#5 - UpDayDownDay (Alternate-Day Fasting)

The easiest of all the intermittent fasting methods, the Alternate-Day Fasting or the UpDayDownDay method allows you have a minimal amount of food intake in one day and then resort back to normal eating the next day. The practice aims to lower down your calorie intake level by 1/5 of the required normal calorie intake during the day of fasting. Let's say, the regular level of calorie for men is 2,500 and for women is 2,000, in a fasting or down day, the level must be brought down to 500 for men and 400 for women.

To make it easier for you during the "down" period, opt for a meal replacement like protein shakes. You can choose your shakes to be fortified with essential nutrients, and you can take sips of your shakes throughout the day rather than opt for small meals. However, take note that meal replacements like these shakes are advisable only during the first two weeks of your fasting and you are encouraged to eat real meals on your next "down" days. Resort back to regular eating in the next days.

If you are doing some workout regimen, keep your workout days on normal-calorie days as it would be hard for you to hit the gym during low-calorie days.

As this option is all about weight loss, it works perfectly for you if your goal is towards losing weight. People who cut on their calories by 20-25 percent on the average witness a loss of approximately 2 and a half pounds every week as reported on the internet.

This method of intermittent fasting is easy to follow, and there's always a tendency for you to overindulge on it during the regular day. The trick here to stay aligned is by planning and preparing your meal ahead of time, so you don't have to indulge yourself in an eat-all-you-can or drive-thru food once you're up for the feasting.

#6 –Fast Diet (5:2 Fasting)

The Fast Diet method of intermittent fasting is also known as 5:2. As the name itself implies, you have to undergo 2 days of fasting and 5 days of regular eating within a week cycle. On your ordinary days, you won't be worrying about your calorie intake, but on the rest of the week (2 days fast days), you need to reduce your calories, e.g., 500 for women and 600 for men. With these 2 days of your choice every week, it is easier to comply with this kind of health regimen though it could take longer losing weight this way compared to the rest of intermittent fasting methods.

#7 – Daniel Fast

The Daniel Fast is a 28-day fast that combines spiritual belief and nutrition through the unlimited intake of whole, non-processed foods. This method of fasting is popular among Christian believers as it is based on the Biblical foundation as described in the Book of Daniel. (Daniel 1-10). Rather than restricting calorie intake or focusing on weight loss, Daniel Fast limits the type of food consumed to increase the quality of nutrient intake.

Although more of a religious orientation, scientific research supports the Daniel Fast. According to the T. Collin Campbell Center for Nutrition Studies, researchers reveal that those people with cardiovascular disease or metabolic dysfunction experienced an improvement when they implemented the dietary habits of the fast.

Key Takeaways:

- Knowing what you will encounter during intermittent fasting, as well as choosing the best fasting method for your lifestyle will ensure success.

- Slow is the best way to go if you are new to fasting. Buffer your journey to prevent and lessen detoxification and keto-flu symptoms.

- You can slowly ease into fasting by doing a -Day Fruit or Juice Fast, and then try the Leangains Method (16:8 Fasting) or do a 1-day water fast for a period.

- When your body has eventually adjusted to the fasting state, choose the best fasting method that is most comfortable for you, which includes Leangains Method (16:8 Fasting), Eat Stop Eat (24-Hour Fasting), The Warrior Diet (20/4 Diet), Fat Loss Forever, UpDayDownDay (Alternate-Day Fasting), Fast Diet (5:2 Fasting), and Daniel Fast.

Chapter 5: Successfully Transitioning into a Healthier You

Intermittent fasting and caloric restriction is a healthy change. During your transition, you will definitely experience hard days. Here are some tips that will make the journey easier.

Prepare for the Detoxification and Ketosis Symptoms

Unless fasting is a regular part of your health routine, you will experience, or many symptoms as your body can concentrate on removing metabolic waste and adjust to become a fat-burning machine from a glucose-fueled system.

Among the many symptoms of fasting, here are the most common ones, along with how you can efficiently deal with them.

Disrupted Sleep Patterns and Fatigue

Fasting stimulates purging of toxins that require more significant workload than typical so that you will feel more tired than usual. It will take at least 3 days for your body to overcome hunger and cravings from old habits and food. Because fasting is limited or complete abstinence of food, except water, it is a great idea to start your practice during the days when you can rest.

Take naps whenever you can and get to bed by 10 pm, making sure to get 8 hours of sleep every night. Your body works more efficiently at cleansing and repairing itself while you are sleeping. Stick to moderate or light exercise routines. Avoid stress, whether mental, emotional, or physical because they are counterproductive to your fasting.

Headache

Headaches usually happen because you are ditching some bad habits during fasting, such as cutting out processed food and sugar, smoking, caffeine, and alcoholic drinks, which creates withdrawal, causing headaches.

You may also experience dehydration during your fasting period, which also causes headaches. Drink plenty of water, a minimum of about 8 to 10 full glasses of filtered water a day.

Nausea

Changing your lifestyle and diet along with choosing healthier food may cause slight nausea. The best way to avoid this symptom is through proper hydration. Nausea usually will usually pass after a couple of days.

If your symptom advances to vomiting, then your body may be detoxifying too quickly. Your system may try to expel toxins faster than it can eliminate. The best thing to do when this occurs is to change your fasting method.

Detoxification symptoms may progress to ketosis symptoms, including flu-like symptoms, rash, and very rarely vomiting.

Cravings and Hunger

You will also experience hunger, but this will disappear in 1 to 2 days during fasting. Moreover, you will be eliminating a lot of food and drinks that your body consumes typically, such as processed food and sugar, smoking, caffeine, and alcoholic beverages. Reducing or eliminating them will most definitely trigger cravings to those areas you have removed and changed. This symptom will continue longer than hunger. When they flare up, drinking water will decrease these symptoms.

Stay Hydrated

Water will help you keep going while you are in your fasting period. It also helps you burn fats and boost your metabolism.

Prefer Overnight Fasting

When most of your fasting hours occur during the night, it is easier for you to get through it. While you hibernate, you won't be thinking of hunger and avoid food cravings.

Transform Your Thinking Process

When you're thinking of fasting as a form of depriving you of food, the more you will crave for it. But if you think of it as just a form of taking a break from eating, the lesser you will feel the pangs of hunger. Therefore, controlling your mindset can help you get through more comfortable with your fasting.

Start When You're Busy

It's better to start your fasting when you're loaded with activities as this will help your mind stay away from thinking about food. When we are thinking about IF, the idea alone will send us thinking more about food.

Hit the Gym

Mixing workout with intermittent fasting will help you optimize the result. Your exercise does not need to be hardcore. Stick with something easy and straightforward like the full-body strength routine. You can do this 2-3 times a week.

Now that you have a clear overview of what's gone trending in health and fitness programs, particularly in intermittent fasting as you have learned all about its drawbacks and benefits, you are free to choose what plan is best for you. While all of them demonstrate to be effective, you must consider your lifestyle while selecting the best option for you to get the best benefit from it.

Lastly, you have to keep in mind that intermittent fasting is never a diet and therefore works well with nearly all kinds of eating program. Meaning, you can get into intermittent fasting whatever your preferences and nutritional restrictions are. You can be a Paleo diet fanatic, a strict follower of low carb diet, a hardcore supporter of vegan, Ketogenic, low-fat or any other kind of nutritional plan, and you can easily integrate them with intermittent fasting. Intermittent fasting is a dietary lifestyle that aids you in your goal towards obtaining a healthy, lean, and strong body.

Key Takeaways:

- During your transition from a sugar-fueled system into a fat-burning machine, you will encounter some side effects

- You need to prepare for detoxification and keto-flu symptoms, including disrupted sleep patterns and fatigue, headaches, nausea, and cravings and hunger.

- You can easily prevent and remedy these side effects by staying hydrated, preferring overnight fasting, transforming your thinking process, starting your fast on busy days, and hitting the gym.

Conclusion

Upon reaching the end of your reading of this book, you have enough knowledge and probably have experienced some methods of intermittent fasting. We are hoping that this book has guided you through your decision of what program is best for you depending on several factors. Each one of the readers may have plans of undertaking intermittent fasting with different goals in mind. However, this book had focused primarily on your achieving a successful weight loss while building a healthier and leaner body while generating muscle mass.

Now that we have established that intermittent fasting is the best, quickest, and easiest way to lose weight and build a leaner structure, we are advocating for its long-term practice and execution. Make intermittent a lifetime habit, not just a fad or fashion that you use while it is popular.

Getting into the habit of intermittent fasting will give you long-lasting benefits like a healthy body and integrating it into your lifestyle will secure you away from many health risks associated with deadly illnesses.

Final Words

Thank you again for purchasing this book! I really hope this book is able to help you.

The next step is for you to **join our email newsletter** to receive updates on any upcoming new book releases or promotions. You can sign-up for free and as a bonus, you will also receive our *"7 Fitness Mistakes You Don't Know You're Making"* book! This bonus book breaks down many of the most common fitness mistakes and will demystify many of the complexities and science of getting into shape. Having all this fitness knowledge and science organized into an actionable step-by-step book will help you get started in the right direction in your fitness journey! To join our free email newsletter and grab your free book, please visit the link and signup:

Finally, if you enjoyed this book, then I would like to ask you for a favour, would you be kind enough to leave a review for this book? It would be greatly appreciated!

Thank you and good luck in your journey!

Meal Prep

The Ultimate Beginners Guide to
Quick & Easy Weight Loss Meal
Prepping Recipes - Healthy Clean
Eating To Burn Fat Cookbook + 50
Simple Recipes for Rapid Weight
Loss!

By *Louise Jiannes*

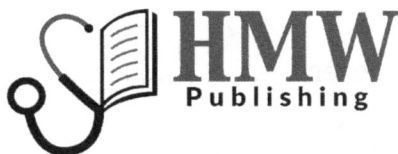

HMW
Publishing

For more great books visit:

HMWPublishing.co

Table of Contents

Introduction

I want to thank you and congratulate you for purchasing the "Meal Prep" book. Every day people are looking for solutions to eat healthily. It is never an easy task to plan meals that are not just tasty but healthy as well. However, because many are so busy in their work or taking care of their children, it becomes difficult for them to prepare healthy and nutritious meals for themselves and their family. Most of the time, they end up buying fast food meals.

Not everyone has the time and budget always to prepare mouth-watering meals in a jiffy. Others for that matter don't know how to make meals in advance because they find it hard to do. But remember, healthy eating has a lot of significant benefits that will not only be good for you but your whole family as well.

Don't fret as you are now holding the key to make healthy meals in advance! This is a great book that will help you get started in preparing nutritious meals for the whole family even if you are busy. In this book, you will learn the basics of food prepping, different foods that you can use to prep your meals in a lot of different ways and more importantly teach you to prepare them the right and nutritious way!

Meal prepping is timesaving, healthy and budget friendly. Aside from that, it is a form of habit that you can include in your daily life. There's no right or wrong way on how to prep your meals, the important thing is that you accumulate the knowledge and make use of it. The possibilities and benefits are truly worthwhile. Start reading and start prepping your meals! Have fun learning and preparing!

Thanks again for purchasing this book, I hope you enjoy it!

Also, before you get started, I recommend you **joining our email newsletter** to receive updates on any upcoming new book releases or promotions. You can sign-up for free, and as a bonus, you will receive a free gift. Our *"Health & Fitness Mistakes You Don't Know You're Making"* book! This book has been written to demystify, expose the top do's and don'ts and to finally equip you with the information you need to get in the best shape of your life. Due to the overwhelming amount of mis-information and lies told by magazines and self-proclaimed "gurus", it's becoming harder and harder to get reliable information to get in shape. As opposed to having to go through dozens of biased, unreliable and un-trustworthy sources to get your health & fitness information.

Everything you need to help you has been broken down in this book for you to easily follow and to immediately get results to achieve your desired fitness goals in the shortest amount of time.

Once again, to join our free email newsletter and to receive a free copy of this valuable book, please visit the link and signup now: **www.hmwpublishing.com/gift**

CHAPTER 1: MEAL PREP 101

When it comes to eating healthy foods, preparation is always the best key to success. One study even suggests that spending your time on cooking and preparing meals is directly linked to having better dietary habits. Meal prepping or meal prep is now becoming a popular craze worldwide. They have been going the main stream, and more people are now doing this kind of food preparation system. People who are engaged on special diets such as Weight Watchers or Paleo have been enjoying the benefits of meal prepping because it can be quite challenging to prepare their dishes especially when they are following a strict diet.

Meal prep can be different from one person to another. Hence it is essential that you will find a schedule that will work well for you and what types of food you love. But first let me show you how meal prepping has become a life changer:

- **Saves time:** the primary benefit of meal prepping is to save time. It enables you to eat healthy during the week without the hassle of preparing it for long hours. It is hard to stare endlessly in front of your refrigerator not knowing what food to make for your family. Knowing efficient meal prep can quickly help you prepare meals in a jiffy plus it will lessen the time that you need to go to supermarket just to buy your meal for the day.

- **Saves money:** some people think that to eat healthily, you have to spend a considerable amount of money. Meal prepping will prove them wrong! On the contrary, meal prepping will help save you some money because you will be able to buy bulk items and lets you utilize your freezer well. Do not be afraid to buy fresh herbs or significant amounts of chicken. There are ways to store them for future use.

- **Lets you make healthy food choices:** being busy does not give too much time for you to prepare meals at home hence the reason why most of the time you opt for fast food meals. The good thing about meal prep is that you don't have to go through eating fast food meals every day. You don't need to rely on them as a last minute alternative.

- **Shopping is made more accessible:** helps you become organized and have a list of the things that you need to prepare your meals. Making a list will help avoid buying processed foods, and sugary products that you don't need.

- **Learning portion control:** if you are following a strict diet or simply want to live a healthy life, portion control is equally necessary to be successful in your journey. Since you are already preparing for your meals in advance, you can know what food and how many calories are there in the food that you will be consuming. This will also give you a great insight into what foods are especially good for your health.

- **Adding variety in your meal:** though it may seem that meal-prepping can be quite challenging, according to statistics people who are not planning for their meal have more tendencies to eat the same food over and over again. Meal prepping, on the other hand, enables you to have a great deal of variety in your meals.

These are just some of the benefits that you can achieve once you start prepping ahead for your meals. The beauty of this is that there are no limits and no strict rules. You have the freedom to be creative and try out different meals for your whole family.

The important thing is that you set aside a little time every week to do it. Once you get familiar with the system that works well with you, it would all happen in a breeze.

CHAPTER 2: GETTING STARTED

If you are new to this kind of method, here are a few of the basic things you need to know so that you can plan and get prepping for your meals.

Evaluating your eating habits

You and your families' eating habits may change every week. It will all depend on your work schedule, school activities, travel plans, commitments and another schedule that you may have lined up for the week. Consider these scenarios when making a plan:

- How many meals do you have in a day? Assess the schedule that you and your family have. Have a rough idea of each and everyone's schedule so that you know how many meals you will be preparing for the whole week.

- Time of preparing the meals: if you think that you have a busy schedule in the week to come, consider looking for recipes that are easy to make or can be left out while you are working like slow cooker recipes.

- Mood: food cravings, changes in season can significantly affect your meal prep. There may be times that the food you want to prepare do not have the ingredients available because it is out of season or unavailable. Weather conditions like winter or rainy seasons need hot and warm food so try to be prepared for these kinds of a situation as well.

- Budget: think of products that are on sale and in season. Sometimes produce that is out of season can be a little expensive. So make sure that you have enough budget to carry out your meal preparations.

- A plan by writing them down with the use of a pen and paper or your apps. Jot down your planned meals, and for how many people would that be. Make sure that you also include what you can do with your leftovers.

Choosing your ingredients

Some tips that you could use in selecting some of the fresh ingredients to prepare healthy and nutritious everyday meals:

- *Look for local produce:* depending on your location, it's best to know the local food available in your market. That way, you will be able to plan the meals that you are going to prepare, and you are already familiar with ingredients that are in season in your area.

- *Meat:* Just like with fish, you would want to look for meat that is bright red. Avoid meat that already has a brownish red color. This means that it's no longer fresh. Make sure that you also smell your meat. If it smells bad, chances are, they are already there for quite a long time – don't buy it.

- *Chicken:* Fresh chicken should be pink in color. Do not buy chicken that is already grayish in color and has tears. Like meat and fish, it's essential that they don't have a funky smell. So always make sure to smell them first. For frozen chicken, check for too much blood as they can sometimes be mishandled while packaging. This increases the risk of having a lot of bacterial contamination because they could have been thawed, then frozen a couple of times.

Just a rule of thumb in choosing fresh fruits and veggies, make sure that they don't have molds, holes, brown spots or wrinkled skin. Most fresh fruits and vegetables have vibrant colors, firm and plump. You can differentiate them from the ones that are old and rotten.

Using your herbs and spices

Our food always tastes better when they are not under seasoned. However, you'll enjoy it a lot more if you know how to use herbs and spices. Be sure to season your prepped meals well to add more great flavor!

- Herbs and spices are used to enhance the flavors of our food and not to hide or disguise them. Be selective in using your herb and spice combination. Do not use too many combinations as this would only confuse or change the taste of your dish.

- For immediate release of flavor, crush herbs, like oregano, thyme, basil, in the palm of your hand before using it on your dish. This will wake up the flavors instantly.

- Dried herbs are used best when combined with oil or water because they will be infused a lot faster. Fresh herbs, on the other hand, provide full, bold flavor to your dish. This is also great for garnishing.

Compiling your recipes

Since you are already set on prepping your meals, it's now time to take a look at various recipes that you will prepare. Look for those recipes that are nutritious, healthy and your family will surely enjoy. Create a master list where you can quickly find the recipe that you will prepare. Every time that you try one, be sure to add them to your roster of recipes.

Be creative and adventurous. Look for new recipes that are worth trying and take note of them. Make sure to take note of the nutrition facts so that you will be able to meet the necessary nutrients that you need especially if you are following a specific diet. Take a look at its serving portions as well for they are essential in your meal prep. It will significantly help especially if you will be feeding your whole family. Don't forget to plan on what you will do with the left-overs.

Another good thing about meal prepping is the use of ingredients. You can select recipes that have the same ingredients which help in minimizing the amount you need to buy.

CHAPTER 3: HACKS AND IDEAS

To give you more ideas and tips on proceeding with your meal preparation, here are some excellent hacks you can try out without having to push yourself too hard!

Cook once a week

Find a day where you can take up some time to do some grocery shopping. It would be nice to do some in bulk, so you do not need to go back to the supermarket now and then just to pick something up. This might seem like a time-consuming task, but it would save you a lot of time in the future.

So take a day or even a half just to buy the things you need for cooking then chop those vegetables and meat and get ready to cook. The advantage of this is that you only need to chop once a week, preheat the oven once, and get everything ready. If it would take you around 10 minutes to cut everything you need for a meal, it would only take you about 40 to reduce those you need for 5 meals, so why not do it all today and just keep them in the freezer where they would stay fresh for at least a week.

Not only is this a time saver but electricity saving as well so you might as well consider committing yourself to cooking a batch of food once a week.

Keep it simple

No need to go and make super fancy, 5-star restaurant kind of dishes. Stay within your comfort zone and relax. Cooking is meant to be enjoyed. Do not make your life more complicated than it already is. Just keep it practical and find recipes that you would want to go and you think would enjoy making.

After all, you are trying to simplify your life by planning and preparing your meals ahead so why complicate it all by doing things that are way beyond your scope? Keep it real.

Fill that freezer

Grab those freezer bags you have or maybe some Tupperware you can write on. Store your food on your fridge to keep them from going rancid and remember to keep your fridge fool from time to time so that you do not go hungry and you are prepared for surprise guests that might come to your house.

Put that slow cooker into use

Maybe you are rushing things because you still want to go somewhere else. But keep in mind that cooking is not something to be done in a rush. It is something to be savored and loved. So why don't you put that slow cooker into use and cook some of the food you would like to see juicy, tender and delicious.

Slow cookers give you food that is just right for the taste, full of flavors and nutrition as well. Most food can even cook up to more than 8 hours so you can go to work and leave your cooker to finish cooking by itself.

Mix and match

Be creative with your food, if you seem to be missing something, just look for something else to substitute it with. Cross-utilizing your ingredients are something that an innovative chef would do so try that one out. Think about the endless combinations of food you can create by doing so.

Keep your fridge organized

You know exactly how vital your refrigerator is to you, so you must do your best to take care of it. Make some arrangement with your fridge and place it in a way that would be most convenient for you. Make it pleasing to the eyes and try to arrange it yourself so you would know exactly where anything is.

These are just some of the hacks that you can try out but do not be bound by them. Along with your journey through meal preparation, you are going to find out more hacks and maybe even create some of your own. The possibilities can be endless, and you only need to take the risk to achieve the things you want; so good luck in preparing your meals!

CHAPTER 4: RECIPES

So now that you are all set with your meal prepping, here are some great recipes that you can try out. From breakfast, snacks even mains – there is something in store for you! Get your aprons and let's get cooking!

Quick oatmeal in a jar

Ingredients

- Fruit of your choice (use freeze-dried for natural sweetness; dried blueberries; dried apples, etc.)

- Milk (coconut, cashew or unsweetened almond milk)

- Dry old-fashioned or rolled oats

Directions

- When prepping ahead, use glass jars about a pint size. Place about ½ cup of dry oats at the bottom of the pot first. Do not use steel cut oats. Add on top your fruit combination choice then seal it tightly. Keep in your pantry until ready to consume. This will last for around 10 days.

- When ready to consume: pour a cup of boiling water or milk. Let it sit for around 10 to 20 minutes. Grab spoon and get ready to go!

Baked chicken and sweet potato

Ingredients

- 6 cloves of diced garlic

- 2 tbsps of olive oil

- 1 sweet potato, cut to an inch thick

- 1 ½ diced onion

- 2 cups of carrots, cut to an inch thick

- 1 lb chicken breast, cut to an inch thick

- 1 lb of steamed broccoli

- 1 tsp of rosemary, dried

- ½ cup parmesan

Directions

- Preheat your oven to 375 degrees F.

- Using a large baking pan, combine all the ingredients except the steamed broccoli and parmesan cheese. Season with pepper and salt then bake for around 30-40 minutes or until chicken is cooked well and veggies are also soft.

- Remove from oven then add the broccoli and parmesan. Place on different individual containers and store until ready to consume.

Freezer Make-Ahead Sandwiches

Ingredients

- 6 pieces of large eggs

- 6 pieces of English muffins

- 6 slices of cheddar cheese

- 18 pieces of deli ham, small slices

Directions

- Preheat your oven to about 350 degrees F.

- Grease a large muffin tray and crack each egg on the slot. Pierce the yolk gently and add pepper and salt. Bake for around 10 to 15 minutes until cooked. Remove from slots and let cook.

- Prepare the sandwich by layering first with cheese then about 3 slices of ham. Top with the baked egg then close the sandwich.

- Wrap with plastic wrap then freeze until ready to consume.

- When eating, remove from wrap then microwave for around a minute on low power. Flip then microwave for another minute.

Apple, Almond, and Cranberry Quick Salad

Ingredients

- 2 chicken breasts

- 4 stalks of chopped celery

- 2 chopped apples

- Pepper and garlic salt for seasoning

- ½ cup of almonds, sliced

- 1/3 cup of cranberries, dried

- 6 to 8 cups of mixed greens

- 2 chopped green onions

- For the dressing

- 5 oz of Greek yogurt, plain

- 1 tbsp of honey

- 1 tbsp of shallots, minced

- 2 tbsps of apple cider vinegar

- ½ tsp of poppy seeds

- Pepper and salt

Directions

- To prepare the dressing, mix all of the ingredients and combine well. Adjust taste if necessary. Scoop around 2 to 3 tablespoons of dressing at the bottom of 4 mason jars. Set aside.

- Meanwhile, season the chicken with pepper and garlic salt then cook using a nonstick skillet until it is cooked well. Let cool then cut to serving pieces.

- Divide the ingredients among the mason jars. Layer in these order: celery on top of the dressing, then apples, chicken, almonds, cranberries then green onions and topmost is the lettuce.

- Screw tightly then store inside refrigerator until ready to consumer. This will last for about 3 days.

Tofu and Zucchini Salad

Ingredients

- 2 zucchinis, spiralized

- 1 cup of carrots, diced

- 1 block of cooked tofu, cubed

- ½ cup of pitted cherries

- ½ of onion, diced

For the dressing

- 1 tbsp of tamari

- 1 ½ tsp of garlic

- 2 tbsp of rice wine

- 1 tsp of ginger

- 1 tbsp of sesame oil

- 1 tbsp of peanut butter

Directions

- Drain any excess water from the spiralized noodles.

- Combine carrots, onions, and cherries in a bowl. Meanwhile cooked tofu according to preference.

- Place spiralized noodles in the bowl with combined mixture. Add the cooked tofu.

- Using a jar, mix all dressing ingredients. Combine well. Place the veggie mixture on top then mix well once ready to consume.

Chicken with Veggies

Ingredients

- 3 pieces of chicken breasts, cut to an inch thick

- 1 chopped red onion

- 2 chopped bell peppers

- 2 chopped zucchinis

- 2 cups of broccoli florets

- 2 cloves of minced garlic

- ½ tsp of pepper

- 1 tsp of salt

- ½ tsp of red pepper flakes

- 2 tbsps of olive or avocado oil

- 1 tbsp of Italian dressing

- 2 to 3 cups of brown rice, cooked

Directions

- Preheat your oven to 450 degrees F. line baking tray with parchment paper then set aside.

- Put the veggies and chicken then season with all of the spices evenly. Drizzle with oil then toss lightly.

- Bake for around 15 to20 minutes or until veggies and chicken are cooked.

- Place about half a cup of rice in containers then divides chicken and veggie mixture evenly at the top of the rice. Cover then store in the refrigerator until ready to consume. This will last for around 5 days.

Quinoa Frittata

Ingredients

- ¼ cup of quinoa, dry

- 4 eggs

- ½ cup of water

- 1 cup of cottage cheese

- ¾ cup of diced ham

- 1 ½ cups of cheddar cheese, shredded

- 1 10 ounces pack of frozen spinach, chopped and thawed

Directions

- Cook quinoa in boiling water covered. Reduce heat and simmer for around 10 minutes. Remove from the heat then fluff using fork then let cool.

- Meanwhile, preheat your oven to around 350 degrees F. Spray a round pie plate with nonstick spray.

- Add beaten eggs with the rest of the ingredients on the pie plate. Bake for around 50 minutes or until the sides become brown. Let cool for approximately 10 minutes then cut. You may also keep it in the refrigerator before consuming.

Buttermilk Pancakes

Ingredients

- A teaspoon of baking powder

- A pinch of salt

- A cup of all-purpose flour

- 1 beaten egg

- ½ teaspoon of baking soda

- A teaspoon of honey or raw sugar

- 1 ½ cups of buttermilk

- A tablespoon of melted butter

Directions

- Combine baking powder, salt, baking soda, and flour. Mix in the egg along with the buttermilk then add it to the flour mixture. Stir well until it becomes smooth.

- Add melted butter than sugar.

- Using a size ¼ measuring cup, scoop the batter then fry on a griddle of about 325 to 350 degrees. This will make around 10 pancakes.

- To store and freeze: cool it entirely after it was cooked. Line a baking sheet using a parchment paper then place the pancakes on it without touching one another. Add another layer of the parchment paper then put another pancake until all pancakes are arranged and ready to be frozen.

- Put it in the refrigerator and freeze until it becomes stable. Once ready to use, you can heat it through toaster, microwave or grill.

Chicken Sausage with Spiralized Veggie

Ingredients

- 1 cup of crushed tomatoes, canned

- ½ tsp of Italian seasoning

- ½ tsp of powdered garlic

- ½ tsp of powdered onion

- 1 cup of sugar snap peas

- 14 oz of spiralized yellow squash

- ½ cup of onion, sliced

- 6 oz of cooked Italian chicken sausage, sliced and halved

- 1 tbsp of Parmesan cheese, grated

Directions

- Preheat your oven to 375 degrees F then line a baking tray with aluminum foil sprayed with nonstick spray.

- Meanwhile, combine seasonings and crushed tomatoes. Lay spiralized veggies, onion and snapped peas on the baking tray. Top it with the chicken sausage and crushed tomato mixture. Cover with aluminum foil then seal the edges to form a packet.

- Bake for around 20 minutes or until the veggies become tender. The open packet then transfers to containers if not eating right away.

Breakfast Quesadillas

Ingredients

- A small diced red onions

- 2 tablespoons of olive oil (divided)

- Half cup of frozen or fresh corn kernels

- ½ teaspoon of ground cumin

- ½ teaspoon of salt (divided)

- A clove of minced garlic

- ¼ teaspoon of paprika (smoked)

- 8 large-sized eggs

- A pinch of black pepper

- A tablespoon of milk

- 10 pieces of large flour tortillas

- 1 (15 oz) canned black beans (rinsed and drained)

- ½ cup of salsa (chunky style; add 2 tablespoons more)

- 1 ½ cup of shredded cheese (depends on your preference)

- Greek yogurt, sliced avocado, chunky salsa (this is optional)

Directions

- In a large-sized skillet, add a tablespoon of olive oil over medium heat. Add onions and cook while stirring them occasionally for about 2 minutes. Add the corn, cumin, ¼ teaspoon of salt, garlic and paprika. Cook for about 3-4 minutes then transfer to a bowl. Set it aside.

- Whisk together the milk, eggs and remaining pepper and salt. Place the skillet again over low to medium flame. Add the remaining tablespoon of olive oil. Once hot, add egg mixture and cook for around 3 to 4 minutes while stirring occasionally until it becomes scrambled. Remove from the heat.

- Drain excess water from the bowl of veggie mixture if there are any. Add them to the skillet with the eggs. Add the black beans the combine well. Season to taste.

- In your working station, place a tortilla and spoon about 1/10 of egg mixture on the half side of the tortilla, make sure that you leave a small space to allow folding.

- Top it with cheese, and a tablespoon of salsa then fold the empty half on top of the filling. This should look like a semi-circle. Repeat the same process on the remaining tortilla.

- To cook, add a small amount of oil or cooking spray on a non-stick pan. Place the prepared tortilla and cook around 5 to 6 minutes until both of the sides are browned and cheese melted. Repeat until all tortillas are cooked.

- Cut into triangles then serve hot. This will make 10 quesadillas.

- For make-ahead meals: cook the eggs and veggies as directed then let cool. Assemble them the same way but instead of cooking, wrap each of the quesadilla using a plastic wrap. To prevent it from bending, place them in a container with a flat surface. Put in the freezer until it becomes firm. Once firm, transfer in an airtight container, then store it back in the freezer.

- Once they are ready to be eaten, remove the plastic wrap, warm it in a microwave for about 2-3 minutes until it is thoroughly heated. Another way of heating it is to thaw them first then cook in the skillet as mentioned in the recipe.

Berry-Berry Blue Breakfast Bars

Ingredients

- 1 ½ cup of 100% pure rolled oats

- ¾ cups of almonds (whole)

- ½ cup of blueberries (dried)

- ½ cup of pistachios

- 1/3 cup of flaxseed (ground)

- 1/3 of walnuts

- 1/3 cup of pepitas

- ¼ cup of sunflower seeds

- 1/3 cup of pure honey (you can also use maple syrup)

- ¼ cup of apple sauce (unsweetened)

- 1 cup of almond butter

Directions

- Place wax or parchment paper in an 8x8 baking pan leaving the paper hang over the edges.

- Combine rolled oats, almonds, blueberries, pistachios, flaxseed, walnuts, pepitas and sunflower seeds in a large sized bowl and mixed them all.

- Slowly add the honey and continue to stir lightly. Then add the almond butter and mix them well.

- Place the batter mix in the lined baking pan and press it firmly using the palm of your hands or if you have a mini roller, you can use that as well. Make sure that it's evenly distributed and rolled.

- Freeze for about an hour. Remove from the freezer and slowly lift the paper with the portion of the mixture. Gently peel the paper and slice it diagonally to long bars, this would make at least 8 bars. Cut them in half to create 16 bars. Place them in a resealable bag and put them in the freezer.

- When you are in a hurry, just get a piece and voila! Makes 16 delicious bars.

Chicken and Garlic Lime Kebabs

Ingredients

- ¼ cup of EVOO (extra virgin olive oil)

- 2 cloves of minced garlic

- A teaspoon of pepper

- A teaspoon of salt

- 4 chicken breasts (boneless and skinless cut to 1 ½ inch)

- 1 piece of lime (juiced)

- 1-2 teaspoons of Sriracha (if desired)

- Skewers

Directions

- Combine lime juice, EVOO, pepper, salt, garlic, and Sriracha. Pour over chicken and place it in a Ziploc or resealable bag. Marinate for about 2-8 hours inside the refrigerator.

- Remove the chicken and thread it on the skewers.

- Preheat your grill to medium to high heat.

- Cook chicken for about 10 to 15 minutes. Turn in once in awhile until chicken is cooked thoroughly.

1. To store, place the raw chicken in the freezer. Make sure that your resealable bag is freezer safe. Once ready to cook, thaw first. Servs of 4.

Veggie Taco Salad

Ingredients

For the cilantro and lime dressing

- Juice from a lime

- ½ cup of loosely packed fresh cilantro

- A tablespoon of apple cider vinegar

- A teaspoon of honey

- A pinch of salt

- ¼ cup of Greek yogurt (non-fat and plain)

For the salad

- ½ cup of black beans

- ¼ diced cucumber

- ¼ cup of corn

- 3 cups of mixed greens

- 1 piece of diced roma tomato

- ¼ cup of diced red pepper

- A tablespoon of cheddar cheese (shredded)

- ¼ of diced avocado

Directions

- Prepare the salad dressing by blending the ingredients all together. Pour it into the bottom of your mason jar, about a quart size. Use those wide-mouth jars)

- Layer the ingredients in this order: cucumber, black beans then tomato, corn then the red pepper, mixed greens, avocado and the cheese.

- Cap it tightly with the lid and place on the refrigerator. This can be stored for 5 days. You can also choose to crush a few tortilla chips on top when you eat it.

Baked Fish Sticks

Ingredients

- 1/3 cup of EVOO

- 3 pieces of large eggs

- 3 cups of Panko bread crumbs

- A tablespoon of seafood seasoning

- 2 ½ lbs of tilapia fillets (skinless and cut to inch strips)

- Kosher salt

- Ketchup and coleslaw to serve

Directions

1. Preheat your oven to 450 degrees F. Using a large-sized rimmed baking pan, place the bread crumbs along with the seafood seasoning, half a teaspoon of salt and oil. Toast inside the oven, tossing it once, for about 5-7 minutes or until it becomes golden brown. Transfer to a bowl.

2. Meanwhile, beat eggs with a tablespoon of water. Dip the fish on the eggs and coat it with the toasted bread crumbs. Shake excess crumbs then place it on a baking pan lined with parchment paper.

3. Bake for about 12-15 minutes or until opaque and crispy. Serve it with ketchup or coleslaw if you like.

4. Uncooked fish sticks can be frozen and stored for 3 months. Freeze them first on a baking sheet until it becomes firm. Transfer to freezer bags and keep in refrigerator. Once you are ready to cook, bake frozen for about 18-20 minutes. Serves 8.

Veggie and Grilled Chicken Bowls

Ingredients

- 16 oz of cooked quinoa

- 4 cups of chopped roasted asparagus

- 4 cups of cauliflower (roasted)

- 4 cups of broccoli florets (roasted)

- 16 oz of cooked brown rice

You can also replace the veggies with:

- 4 cups of Brussels sprouts (roasted)

- 4 cups of haricot verts

For the grilled chicken

- A teaspoon of kosher salt

- A teaspoon of ground cumin

- ½ teaspoon of garlic salt

- ½ teaspoon of smoked paprika

- ½ teaspoon of ground pepper

- 2 pieces of lime

- 3-4 pieces of medium sized chicken breasts (boneless)

Directions

1. To prepare the chicken: Preheat your grill. Combine pepper, salt, paprika, cumin and the garlic salt in a bowl. Pour them over the chicken and place it in a Ziploc or resealable bag. Squeeze the juice of lime inside and marinade for about 1 to 5 hours. You can also grill it immediately. Spray some cooking spray on the grill and cook chicken for about 5 to 6 minutes on each side or until chicken is cooked thoroughly. Let rest for about 10 minutes. Slice chicken thinly and squeeze some more lime juice on top of the chicken.

2. To prepare your veggie bowls, get containers that have the same size. Place ¼ cup of quinoa and rice on each of the containers. Top it with 1 ½ cups of roasted veggies then add in about ½ cup of sliced chicken. Store in the refrigerator and reheat when ready to eat. You can add a low-fat dressing, salsa or hot sauce of choice once heated. Serves 8.

3. In roasting your veggies, place on a large sized baking sheet then drizzle it with EVOO and season to taste with pepper and salt. Cook in your oven over a 375 degrees F until it becomes tender.

Orange Chicken

Ingredients

- Juice of 3 oranges

- 3 tablespoons of fat, preferably coconut oil

- 1 teaspoon of fresh ginger

- Zest from 1 orange

- 1 teaspoon of chili garlic sauce

- 3 tablespoon of coconut aminos, Note: you can substitute with wheat-free soy sauce

- 1 pound of chicken breast, already cut into bite-size pieces

Directions

1. Combine the zest, orange juice, coconut aminos, ginger, and chili garlic sauce in medium size sauce pot over medium heat. Let it simmer for a while.

2. While letting the first ingredients to simmer, heat 3 tablespoons of fat in a sauté

pan over medium-high heat. Add all the chicken breast and let it cook until the color becomes brown and a crust has already formed in each chicken piece.

3. You can now add the chicken to the sauce pot you have prepared a while ago and stir for it to absorb the orange goodness of the orange sauce. You can also let it cool down for a while (at least for 30 minutes) and then preserve it in the freezer. Just reheat in the oven if you are now ready to eat. Serves 4-6.

4. Note: if you are not satisfied with the orange taste, try adding more zest until the desired flavor is attained.

Burrito Bowl

Ingredients

For quinoa:

- 2 cups of water

- ½ teaspoon of salt

- 1/4cup of fresh cilantro (chopped)

- Zest and juice of a lime

- A cup of quinoa

For chicken

- 2 teaspoons of sea salt

- 2 pieces of large-sized chicken

- A tablespoon of ghee or coconut oil

Other ingredients

- 2 pieces of bacon (if desired)

- A large sized sweet potato (washed and cut to half an inch cube)

- A tablespoon of bacon fat (you can also use coconut oil)

- ¾ cup of shredded cheese

- 5 tablespoons of Greek yogurt (plain)

- 3 cups of chopped lettuce

- ½ cup of fresh cilantro

Directions

1. To prepare the quinoa: add water, salt, and quinoa in a pot and bring to boil. Cook and cover for about 20 to 25 minutes or until it becomes fluffy and soft. Let cool and set aside. Once cooled, add lime juice and zest then the ¼ cup of cilantro. Stir to combine well. Add additional lime and adjust taste according to liking.

2. To prepare the chicken: pat dries the chicken breast and season each side with salt. Using a large-sized pan heat over medium to high heat. Cook chicken around 4 minutes on each of its side or until it

becomes brown. Let cool and cut chicken into small chunks. Set aside.

3. Cook the bacon until crispy. Reserve the oil and use it to cook the sweet potatoes. Sear and stir every 3 to 5 minutes. Turn heat to low and continue cooking sweet potatoes until it becomes fork tender. Cool and set aside.

4. To assemble your burrito bowl: once all of the ingredients are cooled, add a tablespoon of Greek yogurt at the bottom of the jar. Top it with around 2 tablespoons of cooked sweet potatoes. Then top it with 3 to 4 tablespoons of the quinoa mixture and layer it with cheese, then a little of crumbled bacon then chicken. Fill it up with salad greens and top it with chopped cilantro before closing lid. Can make at least 5 salad jars.

Freezer-Friendly meatballs

Ingredients

- 1 sprig fresh rosemary, minced

- 2 garlic cloves, minced

- 1 long sprig fresh oregano, minced

- 3 sprigs fresh thyme, minced

- ½ small yellow onion, already chopped

- ¼ cup flat leaf parsley, already chopped

- 2 medium-sized eggs, already whisked

- ½ cup of almond meal

- Black pepper

- 1 teaspoon of red pepper flakes

- ½ cup of parmesan, already finely shredded

- ¼ cup of cream, Note: this is optional.

- ¼ cup of bacon fat

- 1 pound of ground beef

Directions

1. In a medium-sized bowl mix all the ingredients (except the bacon fat) until they are all combined. Using your bare hands, roll and make meatballs. Tip: you can freely turn them into your desired sized but is much better to make them medium in size to cook better.

2. Over medium to medium-high heat, heat the bacon fat in a sauté pan and wait until it's hot enough. You can now add the meatballs and let them fry for about 7 minutes or wait until the bottom is already brown.

3. After cooking on one side, turn the meatballs on the opposite side for the other hand to cook. Wait until that side is also browned. This will take for about another 7 minutes. Put the meatballs on a plate after being cooked. Serve and enjoy! And of course, let the others cool down first and

freeze them for you eat them on any other day.

4. You can cut one meatball in the center and see if it's fully cooked on the inside. If not, just turn the heat to low and let it stay for a few more minutes. It's also inevitable that you'll be able to make many meatball pieces and you can't cook them all at once. The trick is to cook them in batches, and the put the prepared quantities in a warm oven (to keep it hot) while the other batch is fried. This recipe makes about 30 meatballs.

Fennel and Sausage Ragu

Ingredients

- 6 cloves of garlic (minced)

- 2 small white onions (diced)

- 2 small fennel bulbs (diced)

- 2 (32 oz) diced tomatoes, include its juices

- 1 (15 oz) canned tomato puree

- A pound of hot Italian sausage

- EVOO

- 1 sprig of rosemary

- Pepper and salt to taste

- Cooked pasta (for serving)

- Grated parmesan cheese (for serving)

Directions

1. Crumble and sauté sausage with olive oil using a deep pan or Dutch oven. Brown sausage for around 10-15 minutes and continue to stir and scrape. Don't worry if it sticks at the bottom of the pan. It will be used as you cook along the way.

2. Add the diced onions, fennel, and minced garlic. Stir well to combine the sausage with the veggies. Turn the heat down and cook veggies with sausage for about 15 minutes. Once the veggies are tender, add canned tomatoes and tomato puree. Stir and simmer on low to medium heat. Add salt, black pepper, and the rosemary sprig. Continue simmering and loosely cover the pan. Take off the lid after an hour and adjust taste according to your liking.

3. Ladle a good amount of ragu over your cooked pasta and sprinkle it with cheese and fennel fronds on top. You can

refrigerate this ragu for about 5 days and keep frozen for a few months. Makes about 8 servings

Stir-Fry Frozen Dinners

Ingredients

For the base to be stir-fried:

- A pound of chicken thigh or breast (you can also use other proteins such as tofu, beef or pork)

- ½ cup of uncooked brown or white rice

- 2 cloves of smashed garlic

- 1 bell pepper (chopped)

- A cup of sugar snap peas (you can also use other veggies)

For the sauce

- 2 tablespoons of dry sherry

- 2 tablespoons of soy sauce

- 2 tablespoons of water (you can also use vegetable or chicken broth)

- A tablespoon of vinegar (rice wine)

- A teaspoon of sesame oil

- A teaspoon of cornstarch (if you want to have thicker sauce)

Directions

1. Prepare rice according to the instructions on the package. Once done, spread rice over a baking pan and let cool. Transfer using a container or freezer bag. Refrigerate and set aside.

2. Add chicken, bay leaf, and garlic to a pit. Add water, making sure that chicken is covered with few inches of water. Poach and cook chicken on medium to high heat. Let it boil. Once boiling, lower the heat then cover the pot and continue to cook for about 10-13 minutes or until chicken is cooked through.

If you are using tofu, it does not need to be pre-cooked.

3. Once the chicken is cooked, cut into uniform slices and transfer on a baking sheet lined with parchment paper. Make sure to leave room for the veggies.

4. Cut the veggies with the same size as the chicken then place them beside the chicken. Freeze chicken and vegetables until it becomes solid for about 4 hours. You can also do it overnight. Once frozen solid, pack them into freezer bags and make sure to press out air as much as possible.

5. Prepare the sauce by whisking together all of the ingredients. Pour them into a freezer bag and be sure that bags don't have leaks or holes. Again, make sure to press out air as much as possible.

6. Pack all the ingredients together: the rice, sauce, chicken, and veggies, in a large sized freezer bag or container. Label them

accordingly and seal it without too much air as possible. They can be stored for 3 months. This serves 2.To heat your stir-fry meal: defrost the sauce first. Transfer rice to a microwaveable container which is covered loosely and heat for around 2 minutes. You can also incorporate the rice while cooking the chicken and veggies in work.

7. Meanwhile, add 2 teaspoons of oil in a large-sized pan. Add chicken and cook for about 4-6 minutes. Add veggies and cook. Stir occasionally until it is warmed through and crisp-tender. Mix the sauce and stir-fry until sauce thickens. Serve on top of the rice.

Mini Parfaits

Ingredients

- 5 teaspoons of honey (clover)

- 1 ¼ cups of Greek yogurt (vanilla)

- 1 ¼ cups of frozen berries

- 5 tablespoons or more of your preferred granola mix

- Mason jars

Directions

1. Divide all the ingredients equally on 5 (4 oz) mason jars. Place the fruit first on the bottom then honey, the granola mix and finish it up with yogurt. Cover with the lid and store in the refrigerator. This can last for around 3-5 days.

Healthy Snack Bin

Ingredients

- Baby carrots

- Red grapes

- Strawberries

- String cheese

- Apples

- Trail mix of your choice

Directions

1. Place all the ingredients in different packages. To keep the berries fresh, rinse them in water and vinegar mixture, 1 part vinegar (either apple cider or white) and ten parts of water. Then place in a freezer package. Store in the refrigerator until ready to consume. The amount of these snack bins will depend on how much you want to prepare and how long you want it to last.

Sesame Crusted Chicken Bowls

Ingredients

- 12 ounces of asparagus, trimmed

- 1 cup of sesame seeds

- ½ tsp of powdered garlic

- 2 cups of cooked quinoa

- 3 bells peppers, cut to strips

- 1 lb of chicken tenders

- 3 tbsps of olive oil

- Pepper and salt for tasting

- Sesame seeds

- Red pepper flakes, optional

Directions

1. Heat a teaspoon of oil then cooks bell pepper for around 3 to 4 minutes. Set aside.

2. Cook the asparagus in the same pan the season with pepper, powdered garlic, and salt. Cook for around 5 minutes or until tender and bright green. Set aside.

3. Meanwhile, season chicken tenders with pepper, salt, powdered garlic, and oil. Coat firmly with the sesame seeds.

4. Using the same pan once again, add more oil if needed then cook chicken tenders for around 4 to 5 minutes on each of the sides.

5. Assemble the food in separate containers by dividing the quinoa then add chicken, asparagus, and bell pepper alongside. Store in the refrigerator for about four days.

Chicken Chipotle Chili

Ingredients

- 4 cloves of minced garlic

- 2 lbs of chicken breasts (boneless and skinless)

- 2 tbsps of olive oil

- 1 (12 oz) beer

- 1 can of (14 oz) diced tomatoes

- 1 can of (14 oz) black beans

- 1 can of (14 oz) kidney beans

- 1 tbsp of cumin, ground

- 3 pcs of minced chipotle peppers (adobo sauce)

- 1 tbsp of powdered chili

- ¼ cup of Masa Harina

- 1 juice of a lime

- Cilantro and lime wedges for serving

- Cheddar cheese, grated

- Sour cream

Directions

1. Heat olive and sauté garlic and the onions. Cook until soft. Add in chicken then cook until browned lightly. Add three-fourths of the beer and reserve the other. Cook for a bit more than reducing.

2. Add chipotle, powdered chili, tomatoes, salt and cumin. Stir in to combine. Cover and cook for about an hour.

3. Meanwhile, mix the masa harina with the rest of beer then stir until it makes a paste. Add the chili then lime juice. Cook for an additional 10 minutes or until the sauce becomes thick. Serve with the cilantro, cheese, sour cream and lime.

Baked Zucchini Snack Chips

Ingredients

- 1 piece of large zucchini

- Kosher salt

- 2 tbsp of salt

Directions

1. Preheat your oven to 225 degrees F.

2. Line 2 baking trays.

3. Slice zucchini with about 1-2 inch in thickness. Place on paper towels and try to squeeze excess liquid to help cook the zucchini a little faster.

4. Place on the baking tray. Do not crowd. Brush each chip with oil then season with a bit of salt. Avoid over seasoning because it might taste salty.

5. Bake for around 2 or more hours or until they are crisp and not soggy. Let cool. Then keep in airtight containers for approximately 3 days only.

Peach Melba Ref Oatmeal

Ingredients

- 1/3 cup of skim milk

- 1 tsp of chia seeds, dried

- ¼ cup of rolled oats, uncooked

- ¼ cup of Greek yogurt, non-fat

- 2 tbsps of raspberry jam

- ¼ tsp of vanilla extract

- ¼ cup of chopped peaches

Directions

1. Using a mason jar, add milk, yogurt, oats, vanilla extract, jam and chia seeds. Cover with the lid and shake well until thoroughly combined. Remove the top then add peaches. Still well.

2. Cover once again then refrigerate overnight or until ready to consume. Serve chilled. This will last for 3 days.

Breakfast Quinoa Bars

Ingredients

- 1 ½ cups of cooked quinoa

- ½ cups of chopped nuts

- 1 cup of whole wheat flour

- 1 tsp of cinnamon

- 2 tbsps of chia seeds

- 1 tsp of baking soda

- 2/3 cups of peanut butter

- 2 eggs

- ½ cup of honey

- 1 tsp of vanilla

- 1/3 cup of chocolate chips (optional)

- 1/3 cup of raisins

- 2/3 cup of applesauce

Directions

1. Combine the quinoa, vanilla, applesauce, peanut butter, eggs, and honey in a bowl. Mix well. Add the remaining ingredients then stir until mixed well.

2. Spoon the mixture on a greased baking tray then bakes for around 20 minutes on a 375 degrees F.

3. Let it cool then cut to bar size. Store in the refrigerator until ready to eat.

Bacon Choco Chip Cookies

Ingredients

- 2 cups of almond flour
- ¼ teaspoon of salt
- ¼ teaspoon of baking soda
- 6 tablespoons of melted coconut oil
- 4 tablespoons of honey
- 2 teaspoon of vanilla extract
- 2 tablespoons of coconut milk
- 4-6 tablespoons of bacon (crumbled and cooked)
- ½ cup of chocolate chips

Directions

1. Preheat your oven to 350 degrees.
2. Meanwhile using a parchment paper, line the cookie tray.
3. Combine almond flour, salt, and baking soda. Mix them well using a fork.

4. In a separate bowl, combine all of the wet ingredients. Make sure that the coconut oil is melted.

5. Mix the dry and wet ingredients and fold in the bacon crumbs gently. Do not over stir. Fold in well enough to be combined thoroughly. This is now your cookie mixture.

6. Form small balls using your hands and place them on the cookie sheet. Bake for about 8-10 minutes or until it becomes brown on top. Store in refrigerator or airtight container until ready to consume.

Nuts and Seeds Granola Bar

Ingredients

- 1 cup of walnuts (raw)
- 1 ½ cups of almonds (raw)
- 1 cup of pumpkin seeds (raw or sprouted)
- ½ cup of sesame and flax seed combo
- 1 cup of shredded coconut (unsweetened)
- 1 teaspoon of cinnamon
- 2 tablespoons of water
- 3 tablespoons of coconut oil
- 1 teaspoon of vanilla extract
- ½ teaspoon of cinnamon (ground)
- ½ teaspoon of kosher salt
- 1 egg (beaten lightly)

Directions

1. Preheat your oven to 300 degrees.
2. Line your baking tray using a parchment paper.
3. Place the walnuts, almonds and pumpkin seeds inside the blender or food processor.

Pulse a few times until it becomes finely chopped. Makes sure not to grind them into a subtle texture.

4. On a large sized mixing bowl, whisk egg white with water until it becomes bubbly and a bit foamy. Add vanilla extract, salt, and cinnamon and whisk well.

5. Pour in the chopped nuts and seeds together with the shredded coconut. Mix well until everything is evenly coated.

6. Spread the mixture evenly on the lined baking pan. Bake for around 40 minutes or until it becomes crispy and golden brown. Stir it twice.

7. Remove from the oven and allow to cool for about 10 minutes. Using your spatula, scrape the granola and release the large clusters. Once cooled, store it in a resealable plastic or airtight glass jar.

8. Serve it on top of coconut yogurt with fruits, or you can add dried fruit.

Spicy Jicama Shoestring Fries

Ingredients:

- 1 piece of large Jicama (spiralized into noodles)
- 2 tablespoons of olive oil for drizzling
- Pinch of salt to taste
- 1 tablespoon of powdered onion
- 2 tablespoons of cayenne pepper
- 2 tablespoons of powdered chili

Directions

1. Preheat your oven to 405 degrees.
2. Place your Jicama noodles on a baking tray and cut them into small sized noodles making them look like shoestring fries.
3. Drizzle them with olive oil and lightly toss to evenly coat the noodles.
4. Season the Jicama noodles with salt, cayenne pepper, powdered onion and powdered chili. Again lightly toss them so that the spices and seasoning will be evenly distributed. Make sure not to

overcrowd the noodles to avoid sticking together.

5. Bake for 15 minutes then turn it over to bake them again for another 10 to minutes or until your preferred crispiness.

6. Store in an airtight container until 3 days.

Breakfast Porridge

Ingredients

- ½ cup of wild or red rice
- ½ cup of oats (choose the steel-cut ones)
- ¼ cup of faro or pearl barley
- ½ cup of wheat cereal or farina
- 1 piece of orange peel (cut to 2-inch slices)
- 1 part of cinnamon stick
- 1-2 tablespoons of brown sugar (choose from dark or light color)
- ¼ teaspoon of salt
- ¼ cup of dried fruit (pick your favorite fruits)
- 5 cups of water
- Chopped nuts, milk or maple syrup to serve (optional)

Directions

1. 12 hours before serving, you can prepare this dish in time for breakfast. Place rice, barley, farina, and oats inside the slow cooker. Mix in cinnamon stick, salt, sugar, 5 cups of water and orange peel. Add also the dried fruit of your choice.

2. Set the slow cooker for the porridge cycle, such that it will be cooked and prepared once you wake up in the morning. If you don't have a porridge cycle, you can cook for about an hour and warm them in the morning.

3. Serve with syrup or milk, top with nuts if you prefer.

Baked Chicken with Sweet Potato

Ingredients

- 6 cloves of diced garlic

- 2 tbsps of olive oil

- 1 large sweet potato, cut to an inch piece

- 2 cups of carrots, chopped to an inch piece

- 1 ½ cup of diced onions

- 1 lb of chicken breast, cut to an inch piece (raw)

- 1 lb of steamed broccoli

- 1 tsp of rosemary, dried

- ½ cup of parmesan

Directions

1. Preheat your oven to 375 degrees F.

2. Using a large baking tray, place garlic, olive oil, sweet potato, onion, carrots, chicken, plus rosemary. Season with a right amount of pepper and salt then bake for around 30

to 40 minutes or until the chicken is cooked thoroughly and the veggies as well.

3. Add broccoli then parmesan. Place into individual containers.

Pear Noodles with Yogurt Parfait

Ingredients

- Greek yogurt (any flavor of your preference)

- 2 pieces of medium pears

- ¾ cup of diced fruits (mix of strawberries, bananas, and blueberries)

- 1 bowl of your favorite granola

Directions

1. Divide the mixed diced fruit into 3 separate mason jars. Top it with the yogurt then put 1/3 cup of granola in each pot.

2. Top the granola with the pear noodles. Refrigerate if you will not consume yet.

Breakfast Casserole

Ingredients

- A bag of 32 ounces of hash brown potatoes (frozen)
- 1 pound of bacon
- 1 piece of diced small onion
- 8 ounces of cheddar cheese sharp (shredded)
- ½ of diced bell pepper (red)
- ½ of diced bell pepper (green)
- 12 eggs
- 1 cup of milk

Directions

1. Slice bacon into small pieces and cook well. Drain excess fat.
2. Add half a bag of hash browns at the bottom of the crockpot then add half of the cooked

bacon, half onions, half of the red and green bell peppers and shredded cheese.

3. Place remaining half of hash browns on top. Followed by the remaining bacon, onions, cheese and the red and green bell peppers.

4. Meanwhile, crack 12 eggs in a bowl and whisk together with the milk. Pour this mixture into the crockpot and add pepper and salt.

5. Cook the mixture for 4 hours on low.

Easy Pea-sy Soup

Ingredients

- ½ cup of fresh parsley (chopped; plus add 8-10 parsley stems more)
- 4 sprigs of thyme
- 1 pound of green split peas (rinsed and picked over)
- 1 sizeable sized leek (use the light green and white part only; halved and sliced thinly)
- 2 stalks of chopped celery
- 2 pieces of carrots (chopped)
- Salt and pepper
- 1 smoked leg of turkey (around 1to 1 ½ pounds)
- ¼ cup of plain yogurt (non-fat)
- ½ cup of frozen peas (thawed)
- Crusty bread to serve (optional)

Directions

1. Tie thyme together with parsley stems using a kitchen string. Place it in the slow cooker. Add leek, split peas, carrots, celery, a teaspoon of salt and half a teaspoon of pepper. Mix them to combine. Add turkey leg plus 7 cups of water then cover.

2. Cook on low for about 6-8 hours or until peas and turkey is tender. Once done, discard the twigs of herb. Discard bone and skin from the turkey then shred its meat.

3. Stir the soup vigorously to break peas and make soup smoother. You can add water if it is too thick for your preference.

4. Add about ¾ of the shredded turkey on the soup. Set aside a few types of meat for garnishing. Add chopped parsley and season with pepper and salt.

5. Ladle soup into serving bowls. Top with thawed green peas and meat. Serve with bread if you want. Serves 1.

Zucchini Salad with Spinach and Avocado Dressing

Ingredients

- ½ cup of edamame shelled

- 1 ½ cups of spiralized zucchini

- ½ cup of red bell pepper, chopped

- ½ cup of celery, sliced

- ½ cup of cherry tomatoes

- 2 tbsps of olives, optional

- ¼ cup of feta cheese, optional

For the dressing

- ½ of avocado

- ½ cup of spinach, packed

- 2 tbsps of Greek yogurt

- 2 tbsps of EVOO

- Juice of a lemon

- Pepper and salt for tasting

Directions

1. Mix all the dressing ingredients using the blender. Pour at the bottom of the mason jar.

2. Add the celery first then peppers, edamame, cheese, tomatoes, feta cheese and olives – following that order.

3. Lastly, put the zucchini noodles. Cover then refrigerate.

4. When ready to eat, shake the jar well and pour on a plate.

Curried Quinoa Salad

Ingredients

- 4 cups of water

- 2 cups of quinoa

- ½ cup of EVOO (extra virgin olive oil)

- 2 tbsps of curry powder

- ¼ cup of apple cider vinegar

- 2 small cloves of minced garlic

- 1 diced cucumber

- 1 lemon, juiced and zested

- 2 diced red bell peppers

- 2 diced green apples

- ¼ cup of thinly sliced basil leaves, sliced thinly

- Salt for tasting

Directions

1. Rinse quinoa then combines it with the curry powder, water, and salt in a large sized pot. Cover then bring to boil. Reduce the heat and continue to simmer for around 18 minutes. Remove from heat then let it stand for 5 more minutes.

2. Meanwhile, combine olive oil, salt, lemon zest and juice, vinegar and garlic. Whisk until combined well. Add the apple, peppers, and cucumber then add the warm quinoa and mix well. Let it sit for awhile until the liquid and flavors are well-absorbed.

3. Add basil then cover. Chill and transfer to plate or bowl when ready to the consumer. Makes around 6-8.

Chicken with Gravy Slow Cooker style

Ingredients

- 4-5 lbs of whole chicken
- 2 tablespoons ghee
- 2 medium-sized onions (chopped)
- 6 cloves peeled garlic
- 1 teaspoon of tomato paste
- ¼ cup of chicken stock
- ¼ cup of white wine
- Your favorite seasoning
- Kosher salt
- Fresh ground pepper

Directions

1. Prepare and chop all your vegetables.

2. Using a large-sized cast iron pan, melt ghee over medium to high heat. Sauté garlic and the onions. Add tomato paste. Cook for about 8-10 minutes and season the veggies with pepper and salt.

3. When all the veggies are lightly brown and soft, deglaze the pan with white wine and transfer everything in your slow cooker.

4. Meanwhile, season your chicken with pepper and salt and your favorite seasoning. Make sure to season them inside and out. Place the chicken, breast facing down inside the cooker. Cook on low heat for about 4-6 hours.

5. Once the cooking is done, take the chicken out and let it sit for about 20 minutes.

6. Take the excess fat on top of the vegetables inside the slow cooker. Using an immersion blender or hand blender, blend thoroughly until the mixture turned to a mouth-watering gravy. Adjust seasoning according to preference.

7. Slice or rip off your chicken using your hand's Place on a serving plate and put gravy on top of a small bowl.

Chia, Ginger and Grapefruit Pudding

Ingredients

For the pudding

- 6 to 7 tbsps of chia seeds

- 1 tsp of grated ginger

- ½ cup of canned coconut milk (full fat)

- 1 ½ cups of nondairy milk (unsweetened)

- 1 tsp of vanilla extract

- 1 to 3 tsp of maple syrup

For the topping

- ¼ cup of toasted coconut flakes, unsweetened

- 2 grapefruits, cut to segments

Directions

1. In a bowl, mix all the ingredients in the pudding. Cover then refrigerate for around 2 hours until it becomes thick. Shake or whisk occasionally. If the dessert seemed to

be thin after 2 hours, add more chia seeds, just 1 tablespoon letting it sit for another hour until it achieves a pudding-like texture.

2. Spoon in individual servings and top it with coconut and grapefruit. Makes about 2 servings.

Spiralized Zucchini with Corn and Tomatoes

Ingredients

- 4 medium size spiralized zucchini

- 2 ears of sweet corn (kernels removed from the cob)

- 1 pint of halved cherry tomatoes

- ½ cup of basil leaves

- ½ cup of Parmesan cheese shaved

- For the dressing

- ¼ cup of olive oil

- ¼ cup of grapeseed oil or any light oil

- ¼ cup of champagne vinegar

- ¼ tsp of sugar

- ½ tsp of kosher salt

- 1 clove of crushed garlic

Directions

1. Combine the corn, tomatoes, and zucchini in a bowl. Set aside.

2. Meanwhile, add all dressing ingredients in a jar and mix well. Add the zucchini mixture on top then place on the refrigerator. When ready to consume, shake well until thoroughly soaked.

3. Transfer to plate then top with cheese and basil. Serve.

Vegetarian Lasagna

Ingredients

- 1 26 oz jar of marinara sauce
- 1 14 ½ oz of canned diced tomatoes
- 1 8 oz pack of no-boil lasagna noodles
- 1 15 oz container of part-skimmed ricotta cheese
- 1 8 oz pack of mozzarella (shredded)
- 1 10 oz package of frozen spinach (thawed, chopped and squeezed to dry)
- 1 cup of veggie crumbles (frozen)

Directions

1. In a medium-sized bowl, combine tomatoes with its juice and marinara sauce.
2. Meanwhile, using a non-stick cooking spray, spray the bottom of the crockpot. Spoon a cup of tomato sauce mixture at the bottom.
3. Arrange ¼ of the noodles over the sauce. Overlap the noodles and make sure to break them to cover much of the sauce.

4. Spoon about ¾ cup of sauce on top of the noodles and top it with a half a cup of ricotta and half a cup of shredded mozzarella. Spread half of the spinach on top of the cheese.

5. Repeat doing the same process, twice beginning with the noodles. Once in the middle layer, replace the spinach using the frozen crumbles. Put remaining noodles and top it with the remaining sauce and cheese.

6. Cover and cook for about 2 ½ - 3 hours on low while 1 ½ - 2 hours on high or you can check to see if the noodles are already tender.

Egg and Veggie Cups

Ingredients

- 1 chopped red bell pepper

- 4 chopped green onions, use both white and green parts

- 8 eggs

- 1 tbsp of olive oil

- 1 chopped orange bell pepper

- Pepper and salt for tasting

Directions

1. Preheat your oven to about 350 degrees F.

2. Heat olive oil in large pan. Add the bell peppers, salt, and green onion. Sauté until veggies for around 5 to 7 minutes or until they are tender and soft. Remove and let cool.

3. Whisk together eggs and salt. Add sautéed veggies then mix well. Place mixture on greased muffin pans just enough to fill.

4. Bake for around 20 minutes or until it becomes puffy,

5. Remove from oven then let it cool. Serve, or it can be kept in the refrigerator in a sealed container for about 4 days. Makes about 12 egg and veggie cups.

Pecan, Cranberry and Orange Granola

Ingredients

- ¼ cup of orange juice

- 1 ½ cups of rice Krispies cereals

- 1 tsp of orange zest

- 1 ½ cups of old-fashioned oats

- ½ tbsp of oil

- 1 lightly beaten egg white

- 2 tbsps of maple syrup

- 2 tbsps of chopped pecans

- 3 tbsps of cranberries, dried

Directions

1. Preheat your oven to 350 degrees F then coat a square baking tray with non-stick spray.

2. Combine the oats with rice Krispies in a large sized bowl. Using another bowl, whisk the orange juice, oil, egg white, maple syrup

and orange zest. Pour in the cereal then stir with the spatula until it is coated evenly.

3. Spread on the baking tray and bake for around 40 to 45 minutes in the oven with 350 degrees F. Stir the mixture every 15 minutes or until it becomes crunchy and golden. Be sure to stir the granola to avoid getting burnt. Cool for around 5 minutes then adds in the pecans and cranberries. Store in a container.

Cashew Milk with Vanilla

Ingredients

- 3 cups of water

- 3 pitted Medjool dates

- 1 cup of raw cashews

- Pinch of salt, optional

- 1 tsp of vanilla extract

Directions

1. Blend in the cashews using a blender until it becomes powdery for around 30 seconds. Do not over blend or it will turn into cashew butter.

2. Add in pitted dates, water, and vanilla extract plus sea salt. Blend it again until it becomes smooth and well combined for around 30 seconds.

3. Store inside the refrigerator in a container that is sealed tightly. This will last for around 5 days.

Energizing Superfood Smoothie

Ingredients

- ½ of avocado

- 1 cup of coconut water

- ½ cup of kale

- ½ cup of tropical fruit (papaya, mango, pineapple or combination)

- ½ cup of spinach

- 1/3 cup of Greek yogurt

- 2 tablespoons of goji berries

- 2 tablespoons of cranberries (dried)

- 1 teaspoon of coconut oil

- 1 teaspoon of maca

- 1 tablespoon of coconut flakes

- 1 teaspoon of wheatgrass powder

- Sweeteners (this is optional; choose from honey, stevia or maple syrup)

Directions

Place all of the ingredients in your blender. Blend well until smooth. Transfer to a glass and enjoy!

Banana, Spinach, and Strawberry

Ingredients

- 2 cups of baby spinach

- 1 large sized banana

- A cup of water

- 4 large sliced strawberries

Directions

Place all of the ingredients in your blender. Blend well until smooth. Transfer to a glass and enjoy!

Kiwi and Banana Smoothie

Ingredients

- ½ cup of water

- 1 medium-sized banana (frozen or fresh)

- A cup of baby spinach

- 2 pieces of kiwi (cut to half and peeled)

- Sea salt

- ½ tablespoon of coconut oil

- A tablespoon of flax seeds or chia seeds

- A tablespoon of coconut flakes or shreds

- Sweeteners like maple syrup, honey or stevia (if desired)

Directions

Place all of the ingredients in your blender. Blend well until smooth. Transfer to a glass and enjoy!

Banana Superfood Smoothie

Ingredients

- 1 medium-sized banana (frozen or fresh)

- A cup of spinach

- 1 ½ cups of almond milk

- ½ cup of strawberries (frozen or fresh)

- 2 tablespoons of Greek yogurt

- ½ cup of mango chunks (frozen or fresh)

- A tablespoon of coconut oil

- A tablespoon of bee pollen

- A tablespoon of chia seed gel or chia seeds

- A cup of kale

- 1 tablespoon of gelatin (you can also use your protein powder)

- 1 tablespoon of hemp seeds

- Any other superfoods that you have (optional)

Directions

Place all of the ingredients in your blender. Blend well until smooth. Transfer to a glass and enjoy!

Orange and Carrot Smoothie

Ingredients

- 2 pieces of peeled clementines

- 4 pieces of shredded carrots (this should be about 2 cups)

- 2/3 cup of Greek yogurt (vanilla)

- A cup of romaine lettuce (chopped)

- ½ cup of ice cubes

Directions

Place all of the ingredients in your blender. Blend well until smooth. Transfer to a glass and enjoy!

Fruity Power Smoothie

Ingredients

- 2 cups of watermelon (cubed and seeded, rinds removed)

- 1 ½ cups of frozen strawberries (unsweetened)

- 1 ½ cup of small-sized cauliflower (florets only)

- 1 (6 oz) Greek yogurt (strawberry flavored)

- 2 tablespoons of strawberry preserves (if desired)

Directions

1. Using a small-sized saucepan cook the cauliflower for around 10 minutes or till it becomes very tender. Drain then rinse with cold water.

2. Place the cooked cauliflower, strawberries, yogurt, watermelon and strawberry preserves if you will use it. Cover then blend

until smooth. Pour into a tall glass. Serve and enjoy!

CONCLUSION

You have finished reading this book. I hope you have learned so much and eventually make meal prepping a habit of your own. You see how beautiful meal prepping is? Take your time and be not afraid to start little by little. Remember that you don't have to prep it all. If you are just a beginner, this will be overwhelming for you. Just try to prepare meals that are good for only a day or two. Don't jump right away into preparing meals all for one week. Once you get comfortable with the process, everything will be easy breezy.

Another reminder is to follow recipes first especially if you are not familiar with some of the ingredients and procedures. This will help in giving you confidence as you go along your meal prep habit. Just focus on preparing the meals ahead of time. Make this book as your guide in your prepping habit. Enjoy and include your family members as well especially your children in making the preparations. This will help them learn the basics at an early age and teach them how to eat healthily.

Finally, give yourself some time to get used to this process. Remember, nothing is learned overnight. There will be some mishaps and mistakes but over time you will learn from them. Do not get discouraged if that happens. Take note that meal prep is about making it easier for you and provide your family a healthy meal every day, not make it stressful for you. So just take it easy. I am confident that you will be able to push through and be successful on this journey.

Again, thank you and have a healthy and happy meal prep journey!

FINAL WORDS

Thank you again for purchasing this book!

I really hope this book is able to help you.

The next step is for you to **join our email newsletter** to receive updates on any upcoming new book releases or promotions. You can sign-up for free and as a bonus, you will also receive our "*7 Fitness Mistakes You Don't Know You're Making*" book! This bonus book breaks down many of the most common fitness mistakes and will demystify many of the complexities and science of getting into shape. Having all this fitness knowledge and science organized into an actionable step-by-step book will help you get started in the right direction in your fitness journey! To join our free email newsletter and grab your free book, please visit the link and signup:

www.hmwpublishing.com/gift

Finally, if you enjoyed this book, then I would like to ask you for a favor, would you be kind enough to leave a review for this book? It would be greatly appreciated!

Thank you and good luck in your journey!

ABOUT THE CO-AUTHOR

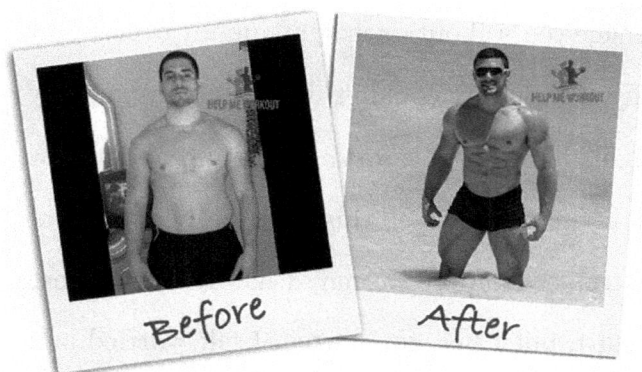

Before   After

My name is George Kaplo; I'm a certified personal trainer from Montreal, Canada. I'll start off by saying I'm not the biggest guy you will ever meet and this has never really been my goal. In fact, I started working out to overcome my biggest insecurity when I was younger, which was my self-confidence. This was due to my height measuring only 5 foot 5 inches (168cm), it pushed me down to attempt anything I ever wanted to achieve in life. You may be going through some challenges right now, or you may simply want to get fit, and I can certainly relate.

For me personally, I was always kind of interested

in the health & fitness world and wanted to gain some muscle due to the numerous bullying in my teenage years about my height and my overweight body. I figured I couldn't do anything about my height, but I sure can do something about how my body looked like. This was the beginning of my transformation journey. I had no idea where to start, but I just got started. I felt worried and afraid at times that other people would make fun of me for doing the exercises the wrong way. I always wished I had a friend that was next to me who was knowledgeable enough to help me get started and "show me the ropes."

After a lot of work, studying and countless trial and errors. Some people began to notice how I was getting more fit and how I was starting to form a keen interest in the topic. This led many friends and new faces to come to me and ask me for fitness advice. At first, it seemed odd when people asked me to help them get in shape. But what kept me going is when they started to see changes in their own body and told me it's the first time that they saw real results! From there, more people kept coming to me, and it made me realize after so much reading and studying in this field that it did help me but it also allowed me to help others. I'm now a fully certified personal trainer and have trained numerous clients to date who have achieved amazing results.

Today, my brother Alex Kaplo (also a Certified Personal Trainer) and I own & operate this publishing venture, where we bring passionate and expert authors to write about health and fitness topics. We also run an online fitness website "HelpMeWorkout.com" and I would love to connect with by inviting you to visit the website on the following page and signing up to our e-mail newsletter (you will even get a free book). Last but not least, if you are in the position I was once in and you want some guidance, don't hesitate and ask... I'll be there to help you out!

Your friend and coach,

George Kaplo
Certified Personal Trainer

Download another book for

Free

I want to thank you for purchasing this book and offer you another book (just as long and valuable as this book), "Health & Fitness Mistakes You Don't Know You're Making", completely free.

Visit the link below to signup and receive it:

www.hmwpublishing.com/gift

In this book, I will break down the most common health & fitness mistakes, you are probably committing right now, and I will reveal how you can easily get in the best shape of your life!

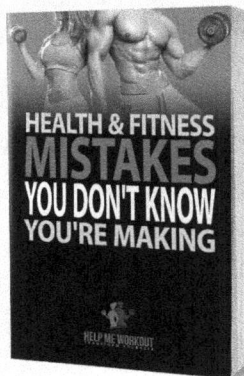

In addition to this valuable gift, you will also have an opportunity to get our new books for free, enter giveaways, and receive other valuable emails from me. Again, visit the link to sign up:

www.hmwpublishing.com/gift

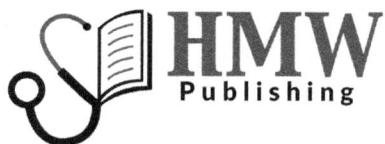

For more great books visit:

HMWPublishing.com